Hidden Treasures

Music and Memory Activities for People With Alzheimer's

by

Cindy Cordrey, MT-BC

First printing 1994 • Second printing 1995
Third printing 1997 • Fourth printing 1998

ElderSong

PUBLICATIONS ◆ INC.

P.O. Box 74
Mt. Airy, Maryland 21771

Cover illustration by Barbara Noll

Printed in the U.S.A.

ISBN 1-879633-18-3

DEDICATION

I dedicate this book to God for...

...His wisdom in giving me wonderful parents, Ron and Yvonne Cheadle

...His love in uniting me with my husband, Neil, who truly is my better half

...His grace for the privilege to be the mother of Cara, Joseph, Emily, and Zachary

...His sovereignty in leading me to my friends at the Evergreen Center, who continually teach me to live one day at a time.

ACKNOWLEDGEMENTS

I want to thank the following for their generosity and diligence in helping me complete this book:

Susan Cheadle - typist

Neil Cordrey - technical writer, encourager, and support person

The editing team - Marie Blackston, Christine Bekowski, Ron Cheadle, Yvonne Cheadle, and Beckie Karras

Barbara Noll - cover design

Also, I want to thank my co-workers at the Evergreen Center for their willingness to help me whenever I have a need:

Elaine, Sue K., Mary S., Mary M., Joanetta, Hazel, Bessie, Margaret, Cami, Sue R., Snookie, Kathy, Terry G., and Dana

CONTENTS

Index to the Song Sheets

INTRODUCTION

It's the start of another day at the Evergreen Center. The clients, mostly senior citizens, begin to arrive, ready to share the activities that have been organized for their time together. Some will participate in a craft while others might chat over coffee and the morning newspaper. It's a warm and friendly atmosphere, especially designed to make everyone feel wanted and comfortable. That's very important to these people, because they all have been diagnosed with Alzheimer's disease.

Alzheimer's disease is an incurable form of dementia or decline in intellectual functioning. It is an irreversible progressive degeneration in a person's brain tissue characterized by plaques and tangles of the neurons in the brain. Symptoms include a gradual loss of abilities in memory, thinking, reasoning, judgment, orientation, and concentration. In the later stages of the disease, the patient becomes totally dependent on others for activities of daily living (eating, dressing, etc.) and highly supervised care becomes essential.

Caring for a family member with Alzheimer's disease is physically and emotionally exhausting. Families find themselves scheduling their activities around the demands of the family member's needs and can eventually find their time consumed by them. To offer families an alternative, organizations like Visiting Nurse Associations (VNA) have developed adult day treatment programs that provide a respite for families and caregivers. The programs usually include remotivational therapies, such as music therapy, in addition to specialized nursing care. Together the therapists and nurses work to create a stimulating and caring environment that encourages participation and socialization, as well as maximum functioning for the Alzheimer's disease client.

The activities in this book were developed with these goals in mind, using music as a motivational tool to stimulate memories and experiences of the Alzheimer's disease client and to provide a means to express confused thoughts and feelings that they may be experiencing that day. I call this "treasure hunting" because so many precious moments have been shared in our times together.

I hope you find this book a useful resource and that you'll try some "treasure hunting" of your own.

Cindy Cordrey, CMT-BC

CHAPTER 1

THE FIRST STEP

The fall of 1987 marks the beginning of my work with Alzheimer's disease clients. Up until that time, I had a vague notion of what the term "Alzheimer's disease" meant—something to do with the loss of short-term memory, right? That seemed easy enough to deal with, so the adventure began.

My first session consisted of eight clients and two program aides in a large room. Everyone sat in a circle of sorts. After introductions I sang "Hello" and away we went.

Looking back on that first session, I wondered why I was hired. At that time I felt I needed to maintain control and that quiet activities in the chairs would suffice. The music seemed appropriate but I was very apprehensive about letting anyone leave their seats.

The following week I arrived early at the center and saw the most remarkable thing. The clients who sat so quietly and passively in their seats the previous week were standing in a circle doing the "Chicken Dance." One by one they danced with the therapeutic recreational specialist as she did the motions. They tried to mirror her motions or improvise on their own. They were laughing, creating, and sharing a special moment together.

Out of my amazement, I realized my conception about the music therapy needs of Alzheimer's disease clients was totally wrong. They needed some sort of order for the confusion and chaos that existed in their everyday world and they needed a way to express laughter, experience fun, and recover the long-ago memories that they treasured the most.

Music could provide this opportunity. For a time, it could allow each of them to be the person he or she used to be before being robbed of personality by the disease. That's what I wanted for my new friends each time we would meet together.

Developing sessions that would meet the diverse needs of the clients proved to be more challenging than I ever imagined. Since I had previously worked with various aged populations with multiple disabilities, I felt I had most of the necessary equipment to be effective, but I needed to find the proper formula so I could make it work for this new venture.

At first, the sessions worked very well because the clients seemed to enjoy doing the activities that were presented in the music session. Everyone appeared to be having a good time together. Gradually, though, I grew frustrated because I was having a problem setting goals for the sessions and the clients. Until then, I had measured success or failure of the music therapy session on whether the clients were showing signs of improvement. It became apparent that no one was meeting this expectation of "improvement" on a consistent basis. In fact, most of the clients were staying the same or even digressing. My self-confidence as a therapist was shaken.

Help came from the center's coordinator. She pointed out to me that "improvement" was an unrealistic goal for this group of people because of the very nature of Alzheimer's disease. Due to the short-term memory loss, it was quite possible and very probable that a client would immediately forget what they had just experienced. What was realistic was to encourage long-term memories and behaviors that were experienced years ago.

This new point of view eventually relieved the frustrations I was experiencing. It also enabled me to see some basic principles that had emerged during the music session (e.g., the importance of structure and the elimination of environmental distractions) which will be explained later in the book. By using these principles (and stacks of creative resource materials), the music sessions began to grow into a shared experience of treasured memories and musical moments.

This book shares some of these moments and ideas with you. I hope they provide a springboard that inspires you to create ideas that will work with your own group(s) and setting.

CHAPTER 2
SETTING UP FOR SUCCESS

ENVIRONMENTAL HAZARDS

Before approaching a music session with any kind of client, it is important to assess the environment and surrounding stimuli present in the room where the session will take place. Eliminate any environmental hazards or distractions (if possible). This should encourage participation, decrease tendencies to wander, and nurture a successful experience.

When dealing with clients with dementia, this becomes even more important because of the distortion of reality caused by the disease. Therefore, it is good to keep these thoughts in mind:

1. **Windows and doors with glass need to be covered so that the client does not become distracted by his/her own reflection.** Some clients become extremely agitated when their reflection appears to be mocking them and they don't understand why.

2. **Avoid having the chairs too close together.** Dementia clients appear to need more personal space and feel "crowded" if spacing is too tight.

3. **Try to avoid as many interruptions as possible.** An interruption can destroy a special moment and, once interrupted, it is usually gone.

4. **Try to ensure that everyone has clear eye contact with you.** Position clients so they are not in front of a column or so far to your side that they only have a side view. Position them so you can meet eye to eye.

5. **Become familiar with the equipment you will be using in the session,** e.g., check the instruments for repairs, cue tapes before the session begins, and determine the correct volume level for each selection.

6. **Match activities to the size of the room where the session will be located.**

7. **Be sensitive to the group's seating arrangement.** Avoid sitting clients together that frequently agitate one another. If this becomes apparent during the session, use the movement of a dance or large motor activity to rearrange the seating.

8. **Try to position the seating arrangement with the clients facing away from the door.** If you have more than one doorway to deal with, position the clients at an angle to eliminate as much movement as possible.

CONCENTRATION BLOCKERS

Dealing with the environmental stimuli is only one of the aspects that need to be evaluated when approaching the music session. Here are some additional thoughts to consider:

1. **Keep activities and directions as simple as possible.** Clients appear to have the greatest amount of success when they are asked to do things one step at a time. Instead of saying, *Let's stand up and make a circle so we can do the "Hokey, Pokey,"* say, *Let's stand up. . .Now, let's hold hands and make a circle. . .Now we are going to do the "Hokey, Pokey."* Simplifying is less overwhelming.

2. **Be flexible!** Every session will contain unplanned interruptions, e.g., a client needing to go to the bathroom, an angry outburst, someone refusing to sit down, or a major medical emergency. Therefore, when it's appropriate, be prepared with alternatives to redirect the remaining clients back to the session. Sometimes the clients can be refocused to the topic prior to the interruption. Other times it will be necessary to abandon your plans and do some group favorites.

3. **Be sensitive to agitated behaviors.** Agitation is a characteristic behavior of Alzheimer's disease clients, usually stemming from confusion and disorientation. However, some agitation can be a direct reaction to something that is being played or sung within the music session. Try to look for a pattern in behavior, e.g., a person who always becomes despondent or agitated during the song "Amazing Grace." It would probably be advisable to avoid it for a time, especially if the person cannot verbalize why that song causes such irritation.

4. **Use the same structure or framework for each music session.** In the book *The 36-Hour Day*, Dr. Peter V. Rabins and Nancy Mace suggest that you "try to establish an environment that allows as much freedom as possible but also offers the structure that confused people need." By establishing a basic routine for the session, the client may eventually learn what to expect next and look forward to that particular activity. I have found in my groups that if I leave out a song from the introduction time, the group members will spontaneously start singing it or ask questions that indicate they know I have left it out.

5. **Be prepared for wanderers.** Encourage clients to sit down, but realize that those clients with sundowner's syndrome will need to wander. I try to include them in organized large motor activities, such as dancing or exercise, accepting their need to wander. (As defined in *Clinical Management of Alzheimer's Disease*, sundowner's syndrome is "characterized by restlessness, excitement, increased confusion, hallucinations and agitation seen in the late afternoon or early evening....")

6. **Use as many nonverbal cues as possible to reinforce your verbal message.** Many dementia clients will respond successfully when clear nonverbal cues are used to demonstrate or pantomime the desired behavior. For example, when asking a client to sit down, hold his hand and "sit down" (squat) next to his chair.

7. **When working with a lower functioning group, phrase any questions asked for yes/no responses.** This will provide the client an opportunity to use a verbal or nonverbal response, eliminating the need for higher communication skills.

8. **Be patient when waiting for clients to respond to a question.** Transmission and communication of thoughts and ideas will take longer for some clients due to the neurological damage caused by the disease. Allowing time for their answers can nonverbally encourage them to keep trying until they are successful.

9. **Maintain as much eye contact as possible.** This will enable you to assess the clients' reactions to activities; it can encourage clients to participate, because they know you are watching them; and eye contact extends attention span.

10. **Select activities that fit the size of your group.** Large groups (over 12 clients) are usually more successful when topics are general and activities include the entire group. Small groups provide an opportunity for activities more individualized to the attending clients.

CHAPTER 3
STRUCTURING A SESSION

Because the need for structure is important for an Alzheimer's client, I follow this general outline for my music sessions (unless other needs preclude it):

    I. Introduction
    II. Movement
    III. Guided instrumental activities
    IV. Target activity
    V. Closing/good-bye

INTRODUCTION

To most Alzheimer's disease clients, every music session is a new experience, something they've never done before. Therefore, I use the beginning of each session to formally greet each client by name, shake hands, and sing "Hello." I also introduce myself and welcome clients to music.

As I am singing hello, I try to establish direct eye contact with every client before I shake his/her hand. I want each one to know what I am doing so that I won't startle or confuse anyone. Sometimes I need to kneel down and look up into someone's face because of the client's physical limitation. Other times, I might have to softly sing hello as I gently approach someone who is sleeping. Whatever way I do it, I want each one to feel welcome.

Following the greeting, I lead three or four songs that the clients enjoy singing (e.g., "You Are My Sunshine," "Oh, What a Beautiful Morning," and "The More We Get Together"). I usually lead the same songs in the same order using brief spoken introductions to tie the songs together. For example, I might say *I'm glad we are together today because...* and then begin singing "You Are My Sunshine," or I'll say *Isn't it a beautiful morning?* and begin singing "Oh, What a Beautiful Morning."

As time has passed, I've discovered two principles about the introduction time. First, the less said between songs, the higher level of participation within the group. It enables you to hook their interest and stimulate group participation, while decreasing the opportunity for confusion.

Second, use the same songs in the same order as often as you can. This routine sequencing becomes a familiar activity that appears to provide a focus for clients, with some actually anticipating the next song. When it is necessary to change the songs during this time, keep the first and last selections the same. Going back to my original example, I might change the opening sequence for the Thanksgiving activity to "Oh, What a Beautiful Morning," "We Gather Together," "Home, Sweet Home," and "The More We Get Together."

MOVEMENT

This time is dedicated to maintaining gross motor skills through dance, exercise, or other movement activities.

Dances, if ambulatory

Encourage clients to stand and participate for as long as they can. Singing a song like "Side by Side" provides a musical motivator for everyone to stand.

1. **"Chicken Dance"**

    The therapist calls out the motions in addition to doing the movements to encourage participation. Motions are repeated four times in each sequence.

    Part 1

    "With a little bit of chirp" - hands raised about eye level, moving fingers up and down on the thumb like a "chirping" bird

    "And a little bit of flap" - flap your arms like "wings" three times

    "And a little bit of tail" - move your hips from side to side three times

    "Clap, clap, clap clap " - four quick claps

    Repeat sequence four times.

    Part 2

    Everyone joins hands and sways back and forth to the interlude. Some clients may be encouraged to step-kick to the steady beat. Repeat Parts 1 and 2 until the end of the music.

2. **"Mexican Hat Dance"**

    Part 1

    Encourage clients to stand and join hands. As the music begins, lead the group toward the middle during the first eight beats, slowly lifting your arms. On the eighth beat, call out "Olé" (if appropriate). During the next eight beats, walk backwards as you slowly lower your arms. Again, on the eighth beat call out "Olé." Repeat the entire sequence.

Part 2

Begin circling the group clockwise for the first 16 beats. (It's amazing how many people automatically circle in this direction!) Circle counterclockwise for the next 16 beats.

Repeat parts 1 and 2 according to your recording.

Variations

- Place a Mexican hat (sombrero) in the middle of the circle to provide a focal point.

- Higher functioning clients may still be able to do the more difficult steps with you that are usually associated with this dance. Pair willing program aides with a client to reduce confusion and simplify steps if needed. You also can feature a client as a guest artist. Here are some steps:

  Part 1

  Partners facing each other. Right heel, left heel, right heel, clap. Left heel, right heel, left heel, clap. Repeat entire sequence three more times.

  Part 2

  Link right elbows with partner. Swing clockwise for eight beats and counter-clockwise for eight beats, calling out "Olé" on eighth beat. Repeat.

  Repeat parts 1 and 2 according to your recording.

3. **"Hokey Pokey"**

This dance activity calls out which part of the body to put in or out of the circle. Encourage participation by demonstrating with your body or gently guiding a client by doing motions together. During the interlude, I frequently feature a client to "do" the hokey pokey, or I'll buddy up with a client to share a one-on-one time together.

4. **Square and Folk Dances**

I use dances that are recorded at one tempo, generally have two parts, and have no calls. I usually have the group hold hands and form a circle and then call out the steps when needed. I try to keep the steps simple and usually change directions or steps every 16 beats. Steps include circling to the right, circling to the left, moving in towards the middle, and moving out again. Some of our favorites are "Turkey in the Straw," "Cotton-eyed Joe," "Virginia Reel," "Hava Nagila," and various polkas and German dances.

I have done some of these dances with partners by pairing a client and a program aide or a client and a therapist. These times are limited because of the need for a one-on-one partnership. The steps are called out by the therapist, with a practice time to orient the staff person with the sequencing prior to adding the music. The performance can be done as a featured "event of the day" by inviting other clients and staff outside of the usual music session. It can also be videotaped for future public relations or a rainy day!

5. "Alley Cat"

Encourage clients to form a circle and join hands. Begin music and call out first steps during musical introduction. As you progress through the dance, anticipate changes in steps slightly ahead of when they are needed. Some clients will be more successful in sequencing movements if you sing the calls to the music.

Part 1

Beats 1-8: Right foot tapping in "out/in" pattern

Beats 9-16: Left foot tapping in "out/in" pattern

Beats 17-32: Repeat entire sequence

Beats 33-40: Right foot tapping in "up/down" pattern

Beats 41-48: Left foot tapping in "up/down" pattern

Part 2

Beats 1-32: Encourage clients to sway to the music. Some people may begin clapping to the beat or spontaneously partner off with a fellow client. I try to be sensitive to their needs by reinforcing their creativity and occasionally encourage them to be the leader.

Repeat parts 1 and 2 according to your recording.

6. **Slow Dances**

I tailor this activity according to the needs and abilities of the clients within the group. Some higher functioning clients will be able to successfully dance together with a minimal amount of encouragement. There have been times when two clients share one of those special moments, a piece of their treasure, that enables them to be like they used to be. The music and dance appear to stimulate areas in their being that otherwise lay dormant, helping to bridge some of the gaps left by the disease.

Other clients will need a greater amount of encouragement and supervision. To eliminate as much confusion as possible, I generally assign a program aide to three or four clients and form several small circles around the room. This allows the clients the freedom to move in time to the music in a secure setting.

I generally choose music that has a medium tempo, with a clear beat.

Movement Activities, if in wheelchairs

1. **"Chicken Dance"**

   The therapist sits and calls out the motions (refer back to ambulatory section) while demonstrating to the clients. Occasionally, I will stand in front of specific clients that need to be more focused, to encourage participation.

2. **"Michael, Row the Boat Ashore"**

   Clients "row" boats with a giant stretchband (see page 13) or pantomime the rowing movement.

3. **Balloon Toss**

   Toss a balloon around the group to music and ask clients to hit it back. To help diminish confused or fearful responses, demonstrate with a higher functioning client or program aide how to toss the balloon back and forth. If a client continues to appear fearful of the balloon, he or she may be afraid of being struck in the face. Therefore, instead of tossing it to the person, gently offer the balloon and wait for a response. Many will eventually touch it and participate. Some will not. Thank him/her for trying and move on to the next client.

GUIDED INSTRUMENTAL ACTIVITIES

When I hand out instruments, I usually sing a song like "The More We Play Together" or Raffi's "I'm in the Mood for Singing." To diminish confusion, I briefly demonstrate how to play the instrument before I hand it to the client. This encourages the clients to respond in an appropriate manner by playing along with my song.

I choose maracas, jingle bells, and a log drum for general use. These instruments are easy to play and make a sound with even the slightest movement, enabling the client to experience the vibrotactile stimulation.

Here are two activities:

1. The activity, "Oh Play Along With Me," is an adaptation of Hap Palmer's song "Shake Something." It's a sequential song that enables you to assess spatial awareness. I sit in front of the clients and sing a cappella *Oh, everybody play above your head, above your head,* etc. While I am singing, I play an instrument above my head to encourage participation. The following verses move down the body (e.g., tap your hand, by your knee, by your shoes, all around). I verbally and physically prompt the clients to successfully respond to the song. Also, I encourage the program aides to participate in the activity to reinforce my prompting and give their own encouragement.

This same activity can be used during the playing of "McNamara's Band." Instead of singing the directions of where to play the instrument, I begin playing the instrument above my head and verbally encourage participation. I continue demonstrating where to play the instrument until the song ends. Frequently, I will encourage higher functioning clients to be the leader by kneeling in front of them and saying, *Now Sarah will be the leader of the band.*

2. This activity uses two to three songs that are group favorites and contain a place for a musical pause. For example, I might begin with "Oh! Susanna," inviting everyone to play their instruments and sing along while I accompany them on the guitar. When the part "Oh, Susanna, oh don't you cry for me" is sung, I put an imaginary fermata (hold) over "me" and continue to hold it until I have everyone's attention. We usually share a smile and sometimes a chuckle from someone who suddenly realizes that the music has paused. Then we finish the song.

    Altering the song creates an opportunity to assess the group's ability to focus on the current activity, providing an indicator to the overall functioning level of the group. This assessment enables me to decide what additional songs and/or activities are needed to focus the group on the session's target activity.

TARGET ACTIVITIES

This segment of the session is based on a theme or a shared experience among the clients. It's at this time that we usually go "treasure hunting" into our past and share our memories. Chapter 5 gives 24 target activities that have been successful at the Evergreen Center. Additional activities are given in the next chapter, "Bag of Tricks."

CLOSING/GOOD-BYE

To signal that the session is ending, I sing two or three songs like "Good-bye Ladies" (adapted from Good-night, Ladies"), "Till We Meet Again," and "Side by Side." Then I shake hands and thank everyone for their music as I sing my own good-bye song, "Good-bye, My Friends."

I try to discourage anyone from leaving the group until we've said good-bye because of the possibility that it might be our last one together. For me, it makes the permanent good-byes a little easier to accept.

CHAPTER 4

BAG OF TRICKS

This is a collection of activities that I call my "bag of tricks." They are activities that can be added at any time to redirect clients during environmental or client-related interruptions.

LUMMI STICKS

Lummi or rhythm sticks are wooden dowels, approximately 12 inches long and 3/4 of an inch in diameter. They can be used to focus the group in a controlled activity that encourages gross motor movement and indicates the client's spatial awareness.

Procedure

1. Pass out two lummi sticks to each client. Before handing them to the client, briefly demonstrate how to tap the sticks together.

2. Begin the recording. Use one with a steady beat, of medium tempo, and easy to follow.

3. Sit in front of the clients and direct them to tap the sticks together. Encourage them with verbal and physical prompts as needed.

4. Vary playing locations by tapping above your head, on the floor, to one side, to the other side, and back to the front.

5. You can also go to each client and use one stick to play a duet with him/her. Offer a stick in his/her line of vision and wait for a response. Many will reach out and play on the stick and become more focused on the activity.

GIANT STRETCHBAND

A giant stretchband can be made out of 3/4-inch elastic with the diameter being dependent on the size of your group. You can buy the required amount at a fabric store and sew a seam to connect the two ends together. This will form a big elastic circle that can be used for gross motor movement by shaking, reaching high and low, moving side to side, and rowing back and forth (quick in and out movements).

Procedure

1. Seat clients in a circle.

2. Have everyone hold the stretchband with both hands.

3. Therapist sits with clients.

4. Begin the music.

5. Encourage everyone to follow you in moving the stretchband to the music. Songs that are adaptable are:

    a. "She'll Be Coming Round the Mountain" - Move the stretchband side to side until the word "comes." Stop all motion for four beats. Begin again on the word "coming" and stop every time "comes" is sung.

    b. "Michael, Row the Boat" - Use a rowing motion.

    c. "Moonlight Bay" - Sing the song three times. First time, use a rowing motion; second time, reach up and down; third time, move side to side.

    d. "Yankee Doodle" - Verse 1: short up and down motions directly in front of your chest (like holding reins); chorus: side-to-side movement; verse 2: shaking (quick in/out movements); chorus: side-to-side movement.

GRAB BAG

The grab bag can be a pillowcase or a sack with a drawstring. Before the session, place specific articles in the bag that would stimulate reminiscing on a particular topic. When choosing the items, try to select ones that represent the various life experiences of your clients, i.e., where they grew up, their occupations, size of family, etc.

In the session, ask each client to reach in the bag without looking and choose one object to talk about. Ask, *What does that remind you of?* If a client is reluctant to reach into the bag, reassure them that it's safe by reaching your hand into it.

Examples of items used to stimulate reminiscing can be:

Topic - Memories of Dad

Articles: shaving brush and cup, tie, aftershave, suspenders, pipe, hammer, baseball glove, derby hat or cap, folded newspaper, pocket watch

Topic - Symbols of Christmas

Articles: Christmas card, artificial holly, Christmas tree ornament, candy cane, Christmas stocking, picture of Santa, picture of nativity scene, small artificial Christmas tree, paper snowflake

Topic - School Days

Articles: ruler, slate board, textbook, pencil, chalkboard eraser, inkwell, apple, jump rope, picture of a school bus

I LIKE _____!

Using the melody from "I've Got Rhythm," ask the question *I like _____* to each client as you toss a ball or beanbag to him/her. When the client catches the ball (or beanbag), prompt him/her to fill in the blanks. Example:

I like horseradish
I like singing
I like hot dogs
Who could ask for anything more?

Continue around the circle and involve as many clients as possible.

If a client appears confused, sing his/her name instead of "I" and hand him/her the ball (or beanbag) instead of throwing it. Sometimes I don't use the ball at all. Instead I shake the client's hand or simply sing, *Mary likes _____*, and then I wait for the client's response.

"WHEN YOU'RE SMILING"

Everyone needs special attention. This activity provides a one-on-one experience within the large group setting. Begin by making some comment about the sunshine inside the room: *What happened to all our sunshine inside today?* Then start singing the song "When You're Smiling." Sing to one client for one phrase and then go on to the next.

Example

To Client 1: *When you're smiling...the whole world smiles with you.*
To Client 2: *When you're laughing...the sun comes shining through.*

While singing to the client, frame his/her face with a headless tambourine or empty picture frame. Encourage him/her to smile with you. Go around to every client and end the song with everyone singing the last phrase together.

The song "Smiles" can also be used here. (Lyrics are on page 21.)

"K-K-K Katy"

Sing the song "K-K-K Katy" to each client, substituting his/her name in place of "Katy." Use the word "guy" instead of "girl" when singing to the gentlemen.

Rebus Song Title Cards

Divide a posterboard into thirds and cut. On each strip, illustrate a song title by representing it in pictures. Examples:

1. "You Are My Sunshine"

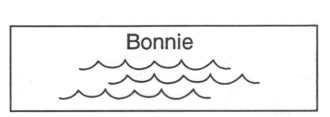

2. "My Bonnie Lies Over the Ocean"

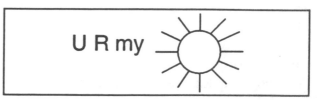

3. "The Bear Went Over the Mountain"

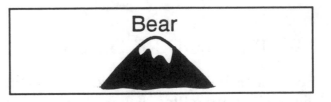

4. "Daisy, Daisy"

5. "When You're Smiling"

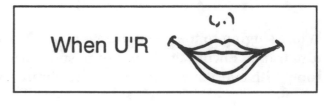

6. "Somewhere Over the Rainbow"

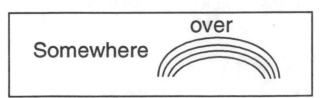

7. "After the Ball"

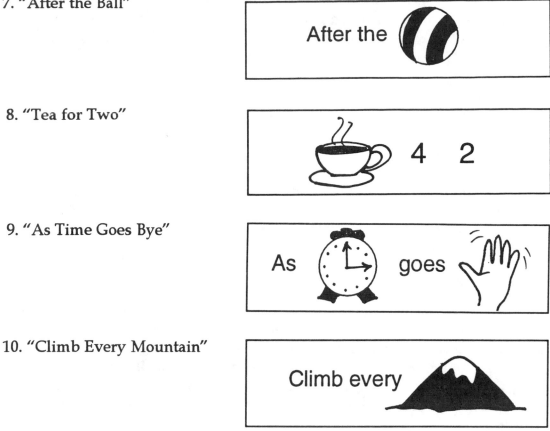

8. "Tea for Two"

9. "As Time Goes Bye"

10. "Climb Every Mountain"

If you invent your own, here are some guidelines:

1. Make all the words horizontal.

2. Give as many clues as possible in sequential order.

3. Put only one title on each card, even if the song has more than one popular title (such as "Daisy" and "Bicycle Built for Two").

4. Use only one or two colors in the illustrations. Too many colors can distract the clients' ability to focus on the content of the illustrations.

FOUR-LEAF CLOVER

This is a picture puzzle based on the song "I'm Looking Over a Four-leaf Clover." I use this to establish eye contact with each client and to focus his/her attention back to the music circle.

Picture Puzzle Preparation

Draw a four-leaf clover on a piece of light green construction paper. Cut the clover out carefully so that it can fit inside the paper like a puzzle. Put the clover aside.

Next, lay the light green sheet (the one with a clover missing from it) on top of a dark green sheet of construction paper. You should see a dark green clover framed in light green. Glue the light green paper on top of the dark green one. Pick up the cutout clover. On each one of its leaves, draw a picture of:

1. Sunshine
2. Rain
3. Roses
4. Somebody you adore

Label each leaf. Now cut the clover into four pieces with a leaf in each piece. Put a small piece of rolled tape on the back of each piece and fit them onto the light green/dark green frame.

Procedure

Begin singing "I'm Looking Over a Four-leaf Clover." Hold up the picture puzzle so that the clients can see it. When you come to the part "one leaf is sunshine" take off the sunshine leaf and hand it to a client. Do the same for remaining leaves. Continue to hold up the picturegram and sing, *I'm looking over a four-leaf clover that I overlooked before.* Ask the clients what appeared on the paper and usually someone will answer correctly. Sing the song through as many times as necessary for each client to hold a clover leaf.

PARACHUTES

Parachutes are colorful and definitely an attention grabber! They are manufactured by several companies and come in different sizes.

I usually keep the motions simple and repetitive so that everyone can have a successful experience.

Procedure

1. Select music that is lively, but not too fast. Folk and ethnic dance music provide a refreshing variety, along with big band and Broadway musical selections.

2. Seat clients in a circle, asking clients to use both hands to hold the parachute. To diminish confusion, place program aides strategically around the circle to assist you with the clients.

3. Warm up the group by having everyone lift the parachute as high as they can, holding it for four counts, and then bringing it down.

4. Rehearse the motions that will be used with the music. Verbally and physically prompt clients as needed.

5. Keep motions simple and repetitive to encourage successful participation. Motions can include:

   a. Slowly lift the parachute above your head.

   b. Shaking - Do quick up/down movements chest high.

   c. Slowly lower the parachute below your knees (if space allows).

   d. Quick upward jerk - I usually use this with higher functioning clients as an ending to the activity or the "pop" for "Pop Goes the Weasel."

   e. Pull and push - Encourage clients on one side of the circle to lean back, pulling the parachute back as well. The opposite side then pulls. Take turns pushing and pulling.

6. Variation - Put one or two balloons in the middle of the parachute. Encourage clients to make them dance by shaking the parachute to the music.

GUITAR DUETS

To add variety to a sing-along, invite a client to play a "duet" on the guitar with you. Ask a client to strum the strings while you finger the chords of a favorite song. Clients can stand next to you and strum, or you can kneel beside those who are seated. Establish eye contact with each as you invite him/her to play and allow the person the opportunity to practice strumming before you include the group.

SILK SCARVES

Silk scarves come in different shapes and sizes, and are easily obtained at fabric stores as silk remnants. When coupled with music and imagery, scarves can provide sensory stimulation in addition to eliciting varied gross motor and social responses.

Procedure

1. Use colorful silk remnants that are approximately 36 inches square.

2. Before handing out the scarves, hold one up and demonstrate how it can move to represent the desired imagery (e.g., snowflakes, leaves dancing in the wind, etc.).

3. Begin a recording that reinforces the imagery (e.g., "Let it Snow" for snowflakes, "Autumn Leaves" for dancing leaves) and hand a scarf to each client.

4. Encourage reluctant clients to participate by standing or kneeling in front of them, establishing direct eye contact, and inviting them to join you in your movements.

5. Lower functioning clients can be included by softly rubbing the scarf on the client's hand. The client may begin stroking or rubbing the scarf alone, or may enjoy the therapist continuing to use the scarf to provide tactile stimulation.

6. Some of the most interesting responses that I have experienced occurred during our "Hawaiian Luau." I was encouraging everyone to dance their scarf in a side-to-side movement in a "Hawaiian grass skirt" style to a recording of the "Hawaiian Wedding Song." Several clients spontaneously began pairing off. Some began dancing their scarves on their partner's head and arms. Other clients held one scarf between them, each holding one end, swinging it back and forth to the tempo of the music. Another dear lady draped her scarf around her head, holding it together under her chin. When I offered to tie her scarf, she told me to leave her "veil" alone! I began asking her questions about her wedding and she shared a treasured memory with me.

DRUM TALK

This activity can provide any client, verbal or nonverbal, the opportunity to communicate with the therapist. Choose a drum that is easy to hold and provides a good response, even if lightly tapped. I prefer a hand drum.

Procedure

1. Choose a song or chant that has a call-response format. Example:

   Therapist: (spoken or sung) *Play the drum one time!* (Hit the drum once.)
   Client response could be one or more hits.

2. Give each client the opportunity to play the drum with you.

3. Vary the song or chant according to the client's attention span that day.

4. Vary the order of who will be next to play with you. Anticipation appears to keep the attention level higher than predictably following the seating order.

Smiles

There are smiles that make us happy,

There are smiles that make us blue;

There are smiles that steal away the teardrops

As the sunbeams steal away the dew.

There are smiles that have a tender meaning

That the eyes of love alone may see,

And the smiles that fill my life with sunshine

Are the smiles that you give to me.

CHAPTER 5

TREASURE HUNTING: TARGET ACTIVITIES

The majority of the following target activities emphasize orientation and remotivation through the use of reminiscing and music. Some activities promote seasonal awareness, others highlight common experiences once shared by all. Each activity seeks to provide the clients with a means to express confused thoughts and feelings and turn them into positive experiences.

Because each center and client population is unique, activities that have been successful at the Evergreen Center may not work for you. Use these ideas as a springboard for your specific group of personalities and create sessions that fit your situation.

TARGET ACTIVITY 1
What's Cooking?

Goals

1. Stimulate memories of family times and favorite meals.

2. Encourage group participation.

3. Give opportunity to make choices.

Materials Needed

1. Beanbag

2. Cooking utensils:

   large plastic bowls
   various serving spoons
   manual can opener
   manual eggbeater
   rolling pin
   egg timer
   measuring cups and spoons

3. Recording of "Alexander's Ragtime Band"

Activity

1. Focus group by singing two or three songs about family meals or being in the kitchen. Examples:

   "K-K-K-Katy"
   "Someone's in the Kitchen with Dinah"
   "Tea for Two"
   "If I Knew You Were Coming, I'd've Baked a Cake"

2. Encourage clients to reminisce about special meals with their families by asking questions like these: *Did your family get together on certain holidays for a big family meal? Which*

holiday? Did you usually have the same menu each year? Was the table set with the best dishes? Who fixed the meal? Did you help? Did everyone sit down to the table together?

3. Ask the clients, *What is your favorite food?* Begin singing "I like _____" (see page 15 in "Bag of Tricks") and toss a beanbag to each client. Encourage him/her to respond with the name of a favorite food and then toss the beanbag back to you.

4. Discuss what cooking utensils would be used to make some of their favorite foods. Take the basket of cooking utensils and encourage each client to choose one. Ask questions like these: *Do you have a special recipe that you would prepare using this utensil? What is it? Is this utensil like the one you use? If not, what is different about it? Do you give your special recipes to other people?*

5. Have clients use the utensils for a kitchen band. Say something like, *You know what else these utensils can be used for? A kitchen band!* Demonstrate how the spoons, spatulas, etc., can each be used to play as an instrument. Encourage everyone to play along to a recording of "Alexander's Ragtime Band."

6. Ask clients to complete several food pairs. Say the first half of the pair, then wait for a response. Answers may vary. Examples:

    spaghetti and. . .meatballs
    bread and. . .butter
    cream and. . .sugar
    salt and. . .pepper
    pork and. . .beans
    peanut butter and. . .jelly
    meat and. . .potatoes
    lox and. . .bagels
    cake and. . .ice cream
    soup and. . .salad
    macaroni and. . .cheese
    turkey and. . .gravy
    crackers and. . .cheese
    liver and. . .onions
    ketchup and. . .mustard
    pancakes and. . .sausage
    eggs and. . .bacon
    coffee and. . .donuts

7. Ask the clients what they do after a big meal. Try to match some activities to their responses. Examples:

    take a nap - sing "Frére Jacques"
    take a walk - play lummi sticks to "While Strolling Through the Park One Day"
    watch a ball game - toss a balloon to "Take Me Out to the Ball Game"
    play games - do the "Hokey Pokey"

8. End the session by singing "The More We Get Together."

Additional Activities

1. Coordinate with the activity therapist to schedule the clients to plan and prepare a meal on the day of this session. If a whole meal isn't possible, schedule making cookies or another easy recipe.

2. Play Alphabet Foods. List the alphabet vertically along a large sheet of paper. Encourage the clients and support staff to think of a food for every letter of the alphabet.

TARGET ACTIVITY 2
Rainbow of Colors

Goals

1. Give opportunity to make choices by selecting the next client to answer a question.

2. Encourage group participation through playing a game.

3. Encourage the clients to help lead the group in an activity (if appropriate).

Materials Needed

1. Six-inch foam cube with different colored construction paper squares taped on each side. Each construction paper square has a number—either 1, 2, or 3. Each number appears twice on the cube.

2. Trivia questions on colors. (Examples are given on pages 27 and 28.)

   a. Questions can include songs, movie titles, holidays, and famous people that are associated with colors.

   b. Divide the questions into three categories - people, places, or things.

   c. Assign a number to each category: 1 - people, 2 - places, 3 - things.

   d. Coordinate a musical activity for each of the trivia questions.

Activity

1. Encourage the clients to sing "Over the Rainbow."

2. Begin a discussion about colors. Ask questions like these: *Do you have a favorite color? What is it? What was the color of your favorite car? Favorite dress? Wedding dress? Name some of the colors of the rainbow.*

3. Introduce the trivia game about colors.

    a. Pick up the foam die. Demonstrate how to roll it on the floor.

    b. Ask someone to help you by rolling the die (if appropriate).

    c. Ask him/her to tell what number is facing up on the die (if appropriate).

    d. Tell the clients that the number determines what category of questions they will answer - people, places, or things.

    e. Ask the client who read the number on the cube to answer a corresponding question.

    f. If a client has trouble answering a question, prompt him/her by humming the melody of the song or singing the melody and the words that are in the song and question.

    g. Do the music activity corresponding with the question. Have the client help with leading the activity (if appropriate).

    h. Help the client who has been assisting you to choose someone to be the next contestant. If the client appears confused, suggest someone, in a way that only needs a yes/no answer, e.g., *Would you like to choose Francis?*

    i. Repeat the procedure for each client.

4. Close the session by singing "I'll Bring You a Rainbow" or "Over the Rainbow."

Color Trivia Game Examples

People

Question - *Who will I give red roses to?* Answer - A blue lady

Activity - Pass out a scarf, either red or blue, to the clients. Encourage them to wave their scarves to a recording of "Red Roses For a Blue Lady." Ask the clients to express how they feel when they are blue through their movements with the scarves. Ask them to express how they feel when they receive a kind gift from someone.

Question - *How tall is the girl with eyes of blue?* Answer - Five foot two

Activity - Ask clients to stand and form a circle (if appropriate). Encourage everyone to join hands and swing their arms and sidestep to a recording of "Five Foot Two, Eyes of Blue."

Question - *You make me happy when skies are what color?* Answer - Grey

Activity - Have clients sing along with you to "You Are My Sunshine."

Question - *What color were your eyes down by the old mill stream?* Answer - Blue

Activity - Ask clients to play rhythm instruments as they sing "Down by the Old Mill Stream."

Question - *I'm dreaming of what color Christmas?* Answer - White

Activity - Toss a balloon to each client to a recording of "White Christmas."

Places

Question - *On what color hill did I find my thrill?* Answer - Blueberry Hill

Activity - Small group and partner dancing to a recording of "Blueberry Hill."

Question - *What color is the little church in the vale?* Answer - Brown

Activity - Sing along to "Little Brown Church in the Vale."

Question - *What valley should you remember?* Answer - Red River Valley

Activity - Clients play the lummi sticks to "Red River Valley."

Question - *What color rose will you find in Texas?* Answer - Yellow

Activity - Group dance to a recording of "The Yellow Rose of Texas."

Things

Question - *What color is the little jug I love?* Answer - Brown

Activity - Have clients do movement sequences with the giant stretchband while singing "Little Brown Jug."

Question - *When you wore a bright yellow tulip, I wore what color rose?* Answer - Red

Activity - Sing along to "When You Wore a Tulip."

Question - *What color is the robin that goes bobbin' along?* Answer - Red

Activity - Have clients play rhythm instruments while singing "When the Red, Red Robin Comes Bob, Bob, Bobbin' Along."

Question - *What color is the old bonnet with the blue ribbons on it?* Answer - Grey

Activity - Sing along to "Put On Your Old Grey Bonnet."

Red River Valley

From this valley they say you are going,
We will miss your bright eyes and sweet smile
For they say you are taking the sunshine
Which has brightened our pathway awhile.

    Come and sit by my side if you love me;
    Do not hasten to bid me adieu,
    But remember the Red River Valley,
    And the girl that has loved you so true.

As you go to your home by the ocean,
May you never forget those sweet hours,
That we spent in the Red River Valley,
And the love we exchanged 'mid the flowers.

    Come and sit by my side if you love me;
    Do not hasten to bid me adieu,
    But remember the Red River Valley,
    And the girl that has loved you so true.

Westward Ho!

Goals

1. Stimulate memories of camping, campfires, and campfire songs.

2. Encourage group participation through dance and songs.

Materials Needed

1. Straw cowboy hat

2. Picture cards for "Hush Little Baby"

    a. Use seven pieces of white card stock (about 8½" x 11" each).

    b. On each piece of card stock, on both sides, draw one of the objects "Papa's gonna buy" for baby. If you're not an artist, look in the library for pictures of these objects and trace them on to tracing paper. Or, make a photocopy of each picture and glue it to the card stock.

       mockingbird
       diamond ring
       looking glass (mirror)
       billy goat
       cart and bull
       Rover (dog)
       horse and cart

    c. Color the pictures or ask higher functioning clients to color them for you (if appropriate).

    d. Laminate each picture card or cover with clear contact paper.

3. Red handkerchiefs (enough for each client and support staff)

4. Tape of western music

5. Song title and activity slips

a. Cut blank paper into one-inch strips.

b. Put the song title on one side and the corresponding activity on the other. Examples:

"She'll Be Comin' Round the Mountain " - Do a giant stretchband activity (see page 13).

"Hush Little Baby" - Sing the song (lyrics are on page 34). As you name something "Papa's gonna buy," hand the picture card to a client to hold. After all the cards are distributed, sing the song again, encouraging the clients to feature their card when it's sung in the song.

"Amazing Grace" - Sing along.

"Battle Hymn of the Republic" - Ask clients to wave small American flags while singing the song.

"Pop Goes the Weasel" - Put a small balloon in the center of a parachute. Encourage clients to lift the parachute when singing the "pop."

"Polly Wolly Doodle" - Clients sing and play rhythm instruments.

"Whistle While You Work" - Encourage clients to whistle and sing.

"Back in the Saddle Again" - Clients play the lummi sticks along with the recording.

Activity

1. Begin focusing the group by singing two or three songs that are usually sung at campfires. Examples:

"Home on the Range"
" Oh! Susanna"
"Down in the Valley"
"On Top of Old Smokey"

Between singing these songs, ask the clients about times they sang around a campfire. Examples:

a. *Did you ever go camping? Where? Were you an adult or child? Who went with you?*

b. *Did you sing any songs around a campfire? What did you sing? Did anyone play an instrument while you sang? What was it?*

c. *What was your favorite part about camping?*

2. Begin a discussion about the pioneers by reading the lyrics of "Ho! Westward Ho!" (words and music by Ossian E. Dodge):

> "The Star of Empire" poets say
> Ho! Westward Ho!
> "Forever takes its onward way!"
> Ho! Westward Ho!
> That this be proven in our land,
> Ho! Westward Ho!
> It seems Jehovah's great command
> Ho! Westward Ho!
> Ho! Westward! Soon the world shall know
> That all is grand in the western land
> Ho! Westward Ho!
>
> Our Pilgrim Fathers sang the song
> Ho! Westward Ho!
> Here Right should triumph over wrong!
> Ho! Westward Ho!
> Still westward many thousands flock,
> Ho! Westward Ho!
> And sing the shout from Plymouth Rock,
> Ho! Westward Ho!
> Ho! Westward! Soon the world shall know
> That all is grand in the western land
> Ho! Westward Ho!

3. Review some of the reasons why a family would leave their homes like the Pilgrims did. Examples:

   a. wanted to own their own homes
   b. a restless spirit
   c. the California gold rush
   d. wanted a fresh start on a new land
   e. religious freedom

4. Talk about how the songs of the frontier helped the pioneers meet the hardships of their daily life. Music was used:

   a. to ease the workload
   b. for evening relaxation around the campfire or fireplace
   c. to play games by
   d. to put babies asleep
   e. to calm cattle herds
   f. to praise the Lord

5. Introduction: *Today we're going to play a musical roundup. Before we begin, I want to give everyone a hankie. Pioneers used to keep a hankie handy to protect themselves from the dust that constantly seemed to be around them.* (Pass out red handkerchiefs to everyone.) Ask the clients to stand in a circle.

    a. Encourage everyone to "shake the dust off their hankies" to "Turkey in the Straw."

    b. Encourage foot tapping or sidestepping (if appropriate).

    c. After everyone has been seated, encourage them to wear their hankies around their necks. (Some clients may want to tuck their hankies up their sleeves—that's fine, too.)

6. Play "Musical Roundup."

    a. Pick up the cowboy hat. Explanation: *The Roundup is similar to playing musical chairs except that we'll pass the hat around the circle while the music is playing.*

    b. When the music stops, the client holding the hat picks out one of the slips of paper with a song and activity on it. (If you have a large group, you might want to limit the activities and just have a sing-along.)

    c. Have the client read the song title and help lead the activity (if appropriate). If not, invite the client to sit by you as you lead the activity.

    d. Place the tape player close to your chair so you can make sure everyone has a turn.

7. Close session by singing "Happy Trails."

Additional Activities for Higher Functioning Clients

Arrange with the dietary staff to serve a western meal; for example, barbecue sandwiches, cornbread, baked beans, and apple cobbler.

Before the session, prepare a chart with the six categories listed in Activity Step 4. Follow the session procedure through to Step 6. During the "Musical Roundup," after a song title has been read, ask the group what category the song would best fit into (of the six categories listed in Step 4). Tape the slip to the category agreed on by the group. Continue on through the session procedures.

Hush, Little Baby

Hush, little baby, don't say a word
Papa's gonna buy you a mockingbird.

And if that mockingbird won't sing,
Papa's gonna buy you a diamond ring.

And if that diamond ring turns to brass,
Papa's gonna buy you a looking glass.

And if that looking glass gets broke,
Papa's gonna buy you a billy goat.

And if that billy goat won't pull,
Papa's gonna buy you a cart and bull.

And if that cart and bull fall over,
Papa's gonna buy you a dog named Rover.

And if that dog named Rover won't bark,
Papa's gonna buy you a horse and cart.

And if that horse and cart fall down,
You'll still be the prettiest baby in town.

Tools of the Trade

Goals

1. Motivate memories associated with clients' occupations.

2. Encourage group participation through games and songs.

Materials Needed

1. Tape with college and military fight songs that represent the institutions your clients attended. Examples:

   a. Air Force - "Falcon Fight Song"
   b. Army - "On, Brave Old Army Team"
   c. Navy - "Anchors Aweigh"
   d. Marines - "The Marines' Hymn"
   e. University of Notre Dame - "Notre Dame Victory March"
   f. Purdue University - "Hail, Purdue"
   g. University of West Virginia - "Hail, West Virginia"

   Resource: "Top Ten College Fight Songs" - distributed by K-Tel Records, 15535 Bedina, Plymouth, MN 55447; 800-328-6640.

2. One pom-pom for each client.

3. Letter cards spelling "Mother." Write each letter of the word "Mother" on a separate piece of card stock. Write the letter on both sides. If there are more than six mothers in the music session, make two sets of cards.

Activity

1. Begin focusing the group by singing "Whistle While You Work." Ask the clients about their early work experiences. Examples: *What was your first job? Did you do jobs around your neighborhood? Did you work before and after school? Was it hard to keep up with your homework? Sing "School Days."*

2. Ask the group how they learned their jobs. Examples: *How did you train for your job? Did you do an apprenticeship? Did your father or a family member teach you a trade? Did you go to college? Did you learn a skill in the military? Which branch of the military did you serve in?*

3. Play "Name that Tune" using recordings of college and military fight songs. Introduction: *Let's see how many of us can identify our college or military academy fight songs. I'll play one recording at a time and when you recognize a fight song, call out its name. You can call out the name of the song even if you didn't go there. While you're listening, let's play some instruments along with the music.* Hand out a rhythm instrument to each client.

    Note: If you have the resources, find out who went to what college or served in the military. (Check clients' charts; talk to staff and family.) Prompt the clients who attended specific institutions as you play their fight song.

    Variation: Use pom-poms in place of the instruments. Talk about attending sporting events where the fight songs were performed.

4. Recognize those jobs that are learned from the "school of hard knocks." Make examples job-specific to those clients in your group. Examples:

    a. Mothers - sing "M-O-T-H-E-R." As you sing each letter of "Mother," hold up a corresponding letter card. Hand it to one of the mothers within the group. Do so with each card. If more than six mothers attend the group, sing the second verse and hand out the additional cards. Leftover cards can be given to support staff or mounted on an easel positioned in front of the group. (Lyrics are on page 38.)

    b. Farmers - Sing "Old MacDonald." Circle dance to "The Farmer and the Cowman" from the musical "Oklahoma."

5. Continue discussion with clients about their jobs by asking them what they did after they got off from work. Examples:

    a. *Did you go home?* Sing "Home Sweet Home."

    b. *Did you go to the racetrack?* Sing and play rhythm instruments to "Camptown Races."

    c. *Did you get together with friends?* Circle dance to "Beer Barrel Polka."

    d. *Did you go see your sweetheart?* Sing "Let Me Call You Sweetheart."

6. Close the session by singing these words to the melody "Taps":

Day is done, gone the sun
From the lake, from the hills, from the sky
All is well, safely rest, God is nigh.

Additional Activity for Higher-functioning Clients

Job Auction (works best with six to eight clients.)

1. Make "occupation bags" before the auction.

   a. Collect tools that are used for a specific occupation. Examples:

   carpenter - hammer, nail apron, pieces of wood, screwdriver

   doctor or nurse - stethoscope, white coat, doctor's bag, thermometer

   baker - apron, baker's hat, icing decorating bag, cookbook

   police officer - police hat, badge, toy police car, toy gun

   car mechanic - car tools, toy car, car air filter

   seamstress - pin cushion, tape measure, pattern

   beautician - curlers, comb and brush, magazine containing fashionable hairstyles

   b. Place objects in a large plastic bag that self-seals.

   c. Lead an activity that can be done by the clients for each occupation. Examples:

   Carpenter: "If I Had a Hammer" recorded by Peter, Paul and Mary. Ask clients to sing and play rhythm instruments to the recording

   Baker: "If I Knew You Were Coming, I'd've Baked a Cake" - group dance

   Beautician: "I'm Gonna Wash That Man Right Out of My Hair" - large motor movement with the parachute

2. Seat clients at a round table. Introduce each bag and talk about what occupation uses these tools. Take the objects out of the bag and encourage the clients to hold them and reminisce about using them. Put the tools back into the bag when everyone is finished.

3. Begin the auction. Introduction: *Today you can choose to do a job you might have always wanted to do. As I hold up each job bag, decide whether you would want to do that job today. If so, hold up your hand.* If more than one person wants the same job, he or she will share the tools from the bag and work together. After everyone has decided what job they want to do, get started.

4. Assign tasks that will be simple to do and provide high levels of success. Examples (if appropriate):

   Carpenter: tighten screws on doors as preventive maintenance
   Baker - place premixed cookie dough on cookie sheets
   Beautician - remove nail polish from fellow clients

M-O-T-H-E-R

M is for the million things she gave me,
O means only that she's growing old,
T is for the tears were shed to save me,
H is for her heart of purest gold,
E is for her eyes, with lovelight shining
R means right and right she'll always be,
Put them all together, they spell MOTHER,
A word that means the world to me.

M is for the mercy she possesses,
O means that I owe her all I own,
T is for her tender sweet caresses
H is for her hands that made a home
E means everything she's done to help me
R means real and regular, you see,
Put them all together, they spell MOTHER,
A word that means the world to me.

TARGET ACTIVITY 5
Turkey 'n' Dressing

Goals

1. Encourage group participation through song and discussion.

2. Stimulate memories of Thanksgiving.

Materials Needed

1. Easel with sheets of paper. Write this verse on the top of the sheet:

> Turkey 'n' dressing
> Turkey 'n' dressing
>
> Pumpkin pie
> Pumpkin pie
>
> Thanksgiving is a holiday
> Thanksgiving is a holiday
>
> Gather round
> Gather round

2. Marker

3. Pictures associated with Thanksgiving. Examples:

   Table set with turkey in the center
   Pilgrims
   Family gathered around the table

Activity

1. Begin focusing the group with two or three songs about Thanksgiving. Examples: "We Gather Together," "Now Thank We All Our God," and "Over the River and Through the Woods." (lyrics are on pages 41 and 42).

2. Lead a discussion about the pictures of Thanksgiving and mount them around the verse on the easel. Some questions could be: *What are these people doing? On what holiday do we give thanks for what we have? Who attended the first Thanksgiving?*

3. Sing the verse on the easel to the tune "Are You Sleeping?" ("Frère Jacques").

   Encourage clients to share their thoughts about Thanksgiving. Jot down these thoughts under the verse and try to shape them into a new verse. Then, sing the two verses. If the group's concentration level is low, sing "Count Your Blessings" and redirect clients to count some of their blessings.

Additional Activities

1. Mount verses on a bulletin board. Ask the clients to provide illustrations for each of the verses, either from magazine clippings, copied pictures, or their own drawings, whichever is appropriate. (This is a table activity.)

2. Write a new verse each year and add it to the previous ones. It will bring back memories for the staff and yourself!

We Gather Together

We gather together to ask the Lord's blessing;
He chastens and hastens His will to make known;
The wicked oppressing now cease from distressing,
Sing praises to His name; He forgets not His own.

Beside us to guide us, our God with us joining,
Ordaining, maintaining His Kingdom divine;
So from the beginning the fight we were winning;
Thou, Lord, wast at our side; all glory be Thine!

Now Thank We All Our God

Now thank we all our God with heart and hands and voices,
Who wondrous things hath done, in whom His world rejoices;
Who, from our mothers' arms, hath blessed us on our way
With countless gifts of love, and still is ours today.

O may this bounteous God through all our life be near us,
With ever joyful hearts and blessed peace to cheer us;
And keep us in His grace, and guide us when perplexed,
And free us from all ills in this world and the next.

All praise and thanks to God the Father now be given,
The Son, and Him who reigns with them in highest heaven,
The one eternal God, whom earth and heaven adore;
For thus it was, is now, and shall be evermore.

Over The River and Through The Woods

Over the river and through the woods,
To grandfather's house we'll go,
The horse knows the way to carry the sleigh
Through the white and drifted snow.
Over the river and through the woods,
Oh, how the wind does blow!
It stings the toes and bites the nose
As over the ground we go.

Over the river and through the woods,
To have a first-rate play,
Hear the bells ring, "ting-a-ling-ding!"
Hurrah for Thanksgiving Day!
Over the river and through the woods,
Trot fast, my dapple gray!
Spring over the ground like a hunting hound!
For this is Thanksgiving Day!

Over the river and through the woods,
And straight through the barnyard gate.
We seem to go extremely slow;
It is so hard to wait!
Over the river and through the woods,
Now grandmother's cap I spy!
Hurrah for the fun! Is the pudding done?
Hurrah for the pumpkin pie!

TARGET ACTIVITY 6
Election Toss-up

Goals

1. Encourage group participation.

2. Encourage participation in group discussion.

3. Give opportunity to make choices.

Materials Needed

1. Recording of patriotic music

2. Fact cards about various presidents (See suggestions below.)

3. Pictures of donkey and elephant

4. Pictures of presidents

5. Two boxes covered with red, white, and blue crepe paper and opened on the top. Inside each box are presidential fact cards, with side 1 of cards facing up. (See suggestions on page 44.)

6. Beanbag

Activity

1. Begin focusing the group by singing various patriotic songs, such as, "This Land is Your Land," "You're A Grand Old Flag," and "America, the Beautiful." (Lyrics for this last song are on page 46.)

2. Show the pictures of the donkey and the elephant and ask what they have to do with voting for a president.

   a. Encourage clients to answer questions about the two main political parties in the United States.

   b. Mount the donkey on one box and the elephant on the other box.

3. Begin the discussion by asking some easy questions about previous presidents. Examples: *Who was the first president?* (George Washington) *Who was president during the Civil War?* (Abraham Lincoln)

4. Place the two boxes in front of each client in turn.

   Review the voting process and weave into the conversation that voting is exercising a choice. Demonstrate that throwing the beanbag into one of the boxes is a choice, too, and that each client will have a chance to "vote" in today's election game.

   Give the beanbag to the client and ask him/her to toss the bag into the box of his/her choice.

   Ask the client to pick a card out of the box chosen. If appropriate, ask the client to read the question on side 1 and answer it (or the group can answer it).

   Give the answer, if needed, and lead the activity that is written below the answer on side 2. If possible, encourage the client to be the leader of the activity chosen.

5. Close the activity by singing "God Bless America."

Card Format Example

Side 1

> Who was the youngest president elected to office?

Side 2

> John Kennedy
>
> Play the lummi sticks to patriotic music.

Presidential fact suggestions:

a. What two presidents were cousins?
   Theodore Roosevelt and Franklin Roosevelt

b. Who was the oldest president voted to office?
   Ronald Reagan

c. What president started the New Deal?
   Harry Truman

d. What president started the March of Dimes Campaign?
   Franklin Roosevelt

e. What president wrote the Declaration of Independence?
   Thomas Jefferson

f. What president was called the "Father of His Country"?
   George Washington

g. What president grew up in Kentucky and Indiana and was called "Honest Abe?"
   Abraham Lincoln

h. In February 1951, the 22nd Amendment to the Constitution was ratified, limiting a president to how many terms in office?
   Two

Activities on the cards can include:

a. Play rhythm instruments or lummi sticks to a patriotic march.

b. Sing the "Star Spangled Banner."

c. Say the "Pledge of Allegiance."

d. Dance to "I'm a Yankee Doodle Dandy."

e. Sing "My Country 'Tis of Thee."

f. March in place to "Yankee Doodle."

America, the Beautiful

O beautiful for spacious skies,
For amber waves of grain,
For purple mountain majesties
Above the fruited plain!
America! America!
God shed his grace on thee
And crown thy good with brotherhood
From sea to shining sea!

O beautiful for patriot dream
That sees beyond the years
Thine alabaster cities gleam
Undimmed by human tears!
America! America!
God shed His grace on thee
And crown thy good with brotherhood
From sea to shining sea!

The Twelve Days of Christmas

Goals

1. Encourage group participation through singing "The Twelve Days of Christmas."

2. Stimulate memories of Christmas.

Materials Needed

1. Pictures of Christmas carolers

2. A pictures for each verse of "The Twelve Days of Christmas" — copy and color a picture for each of the twelve days:

   partridge in a pear tree
   turtledoves
   French hens
   calling birds
   gold rings
   geese a-laying
   swans a-swimming
   maids a-milking
   ladies dancing
   lords a-leaping
   pipers piping
   drummers drumming

3. Tape recording of "The Twelve Days of Christmas"

4. Tape recorder

5. Easel with blank sheet of paper

6. Box wrapped as a Christmas gift

Activity

1. Focus the group by singing two or three traditional Christmas carols.

2. Display the pictures of Christmas carolers for the clients. Let them look at the pictures closely and discuss:

   a. *What are these people doing?*
   b. *Have you ever gone caroling?*
   c. *How did you dress?*
   d. *Do these carolers look like they're having fun?*

3. Invite the clients to have some fun caroling together. Say, *Since caroling looks like something fun to do, let's do it! The song I'm thinking of is "The Twelve Days of Christmas."*

   Give one verse picture to each client and identify the picture. If your group isn't large enough for all the verses, mount the later verses on the easel so everyone can see them. If your group has more than 12 persons, pair up on verses.

   Begin the tape recording. Sing along with the tape and feature the client who is holding the day that is being sung.

   As the song progresses, keep featuring each client whose day is sung. The client with a partridge in a pear tree will be featured 12 times, two turtledoves 11 times, and so on. If you have verse pictures on the easel, point to them as you sing that day.

   After the song is over, collect the verse pictures and ask the clients what gifts they remember receiving from a loved one. Jot down the answers on the easel paper if possible.

4. Pass the Christmas wrapped box from client to client and ask, *What gift would you like to give your family this year?* Jot down the answers on the easel paper.

5. Close the activity with a reflective Christmas carol or song, such as, "I'll Be Home for Christmas," "Let There Be Peace on Earth," or "Silent Night."

Additional Activity

Make Christmas cards from the clients to their families with their suggested "gifts" by their names.

TARGET ACTIVITY 8
A Day at the Beach

Goals

1. Increase seasonal awareness.

2. Encourage group participation.

3. Encourage discussion through topic and stimuli.

Materials Needed

1. Grab bag containing beach items

   Shovel
   Shells
   Suntan lotion
   Sunglasses
   Bucket
   Towel
   Bathing cap
   Bathing suit

2. Basin full of sand

3. Beach ball and parachute

4. Tape recordings of ocean sounds and Hawaiian music

Activity

1. Play recording of ocean sounds. Ask if anyone recognizes the sounds.

2. Begin to focus conversation around a day at the beach.

   a. Ask, *"What will we need to take?"* Encourage each client to "grab" something from the bag to contribute to the list. Ask clients to share memories about the items chosen.

b. Ask, *"How will we get to the beach?"* Songs to sing:

    1. Car - "In My Merry Oldsmobile"
    2. Train - "Chattanooga Choo Choo"
    3. Walking - "Side by Side"

c. Ask, *What will we do when we get there?* Prompt clients with the articles from the grab bag.

    1. Bathing suit - swimming
    2. Suntan lotion - sunbathing on the beach
    3. Shells - shell collecting
    4. Shovel/bucket - making sand castles

d. Song to sing: "My Favorite Things" from the musical "The Sound of Music."

3. Parachute activity to Hawaiian music.

Place the beach ball in the center of the parachute and encourage clients to shake the ball around, toss it in the air, or "bounce" it on the parachute with a quick up/down motion.

4. Take the basin of sand and allow the clients to take turns feeling it in their hands or perhaps on their feet. Sing songs like these:

a. "My Bonnie Lies Over the Ocean"
b. "Michael, Row the Boat Ashore"
c. "Moonlight Bay"

5. Bring everyone "back from the beach" by singing "Side by Side."

TARGET ACTIVITY 9
Signs of Spring

Goals

1. Encourage seasonal awareness.

2. Encourage group participation.

3. Stimulate memories of spring.

Materials Needed

1. Tape recording of the songs "Bye Bye, Blackbird" and "Side by Side"

2. Pictures from magazines, catalogs, etc., of these:

   birds
   people playing baseball
   rain scenes
   flowers
   fish or people fishing
   wedding, sweethearts, etc.

3. Mural paper covering a table (see diagrams on next page)

4. Glue sticks (one for each client)

Activity

1. Arrange clients around the paper-covered table. If you need to move the clients from a circle to the table, try involving everyone in a dance and then guide them to sit around the table as the dance ends.

2. Begin focusing the discussion on what is happening with the weather. Examples:

   a. *Has anyone seen a robin?*
   b. *I noticed that the crocuses were blooming out front.*
   c. *It's getting warmer outside.*

3. Lay out pictures cut from magazines and ask the clients to pick out some pictures that show signs of spring. Go around the table and feature each client with one of his/her selections and sing a song appropriate for it. Encourage clients to share memories of previous springtimes. Examples:

   a. tulips - "When You Wore a Tulip"

   b. roses - "The Yellow Rose of Texas"

   c. birds - "Aura Lee," "Bye Bye, Blackbird," "When the Red, Red Robin Comes Bob, Bob, Bobbin' Along"

   d. sweethearts - "Bicycle Built for Two," "Love's Old Sweet Song," "Let Me Call You Sweetheart"

   e. baseball - "Take Me Out to the Ball Game"

   f. rain - "Singing in the Rain"

   g. weddings - "Put on Your Old Grey Bonnet"

   Between songs, encourage clients to glue their selections on the mural. Have the clients sign their names or sign it for them around the pictures they glued on the mural.

4. After the mural is completed, ask everyone to make a circle (seated or standing, either around the table or in the circle of chairs where they were originally seated). Say, *No matter what the weather, if it's spring, rainy or sunny, we want to be together side by side. Let's sing "Side by Side."*

5. After the session, hang the mural in a location that the clients can see on a daily basis. You might have to cut it in half in order to show everyone's name in an upright position (Diagram 1). Mount the mural on a contrasting background and let everyone enjoy their handiwork (Diagram 2).

Diagram 1

Don	Jean	Mary	John
Mike	Steve	Betty	Linda

Diagram 2

Mike	Steve	Betty	Linda	John	Mary	Jean	Don

TARGET ACTIVITY 10
M-O-T-H-E-R

Goals

1. Encourage group participation.

2. Stimulate memories about the clients' mothers.

Materials Needed

1. Large piece of paper mounted on an easel. Before the session, write the following verse on the paper with a colored marker:

> Have you every met my mother
> My mother, my mother?
> Have you ever met my mother?
> She's a wonderful gal!

   Then write "MOTHER," with a second colored marker, vertically on the large piece of paper under the verse.

2. Markers - two different dark colors

3. Tape recorder and a blank tape

Activity

1. Ask the group to read the word in the middle of the paper (if able to see and/or read).

2. Start singing the tune "Did You Ever See a Lassie?" using the words from the verse on the paper.

3. Ask the clients to talk about their mothers. Try to match comments to words that would begin with the letters M-O-T-H-E-R. Write these words on the paper in the first color so that the letters M, O, T, H, E, and R stand out in the verse.

Example:

> Have you ever met my mother,
> my mother, my mother?
> Have you ever met my mother?
> She's a wonderful gal!
>
> She's a   **M**anager
> She's   **O**verworked
> She's a   **T**eacher
> She's a   **H**elper
> She gives **E**verlasting love
> And I   **R**emember her well

4. Ask the group to sing it through and then make a recording of it. Replay it for the clients to enjoy again. (The first four lines written by clients correspond to the words "go this way and that way," etc. The last two lines use the beginning melody.) Hang the song in a prominent place so the clients can enjoy reading it.

Note: The lyrics to the song "M-O-T-H-E-R" are on page 38.

TARGET ACTIVITY 11

Hats

Great activity for National Hat Day (third Friday in January)

Goals

1. Stimulate memories of hat-wearing events in the clients' lives.

2. Encourage group participation.

Materials Needed

1. Different types of hats (cowboy, colonial, baseball, birthday, winter, sailor, dressy, nurse, straw, etc.)

2. Recording of "Let it Snow," "Mexican Hat Dance," "Easter Parade," "Anchors Away"

3. Giant stretchband

4. Lummi sticks

Activity

1. Put hats in basket.

2. Ask each client to pick a hat and put it on.

3. Discussion questions:

   a. *Have you ever owned a hat like this before? When did you wear it?*
   b. *Do you like wearing a hat?*
   c. *Why do people wear hats?*
   d. *Did you ever wear a hat while you did your job?*

4. Begin "featuring" each hat with a musical activity. When appropriate, ask the wearer to be the leader of the activity. Activity suggestions (not all songs have activities, some are just for singing):

a. cowboy hat - "Home on the Range" (with the giant stretchband)

b. colonial hat - "Yankee Doodle," "My Hat It Has Three Corners"

c. sombrero - "Mexican Hat Dance" (Simplify dance sequences to left/right, right/left, in/out. Refer to page 8.)

d. baseball cap - "Take Me Out to the Ball Game"

e. birthday party hat - "Happy Birthday," "For He's a Jolly Good Fellow"

f. winter hat - "Let It Snow" (dance)

g. army hat - "Pack Up Your Troubles in Your Old Kit Bag"

h. sailor hat - "Anchors Away" (Use lummi sticks to play along to the recording. Encourage gross motor movement throughout the activity. Refer to Bag of Tricks, page 13.)

i. dress hat - "He's Got the Whole World in His Hands," "Amazing Grace"

j. yarmulke - "Hava Nagila"

5. After all the hats have been featured, hold a Hat Parade around the activity circle to the music "Easter Parade." Encourage clients to show off their hats!

Additional Activity

Have clients decorate a hat with some of their favorite things. Purchase small straw hats at a craft store. Decorations can be symbols of occupations, hobbies, or favorite things. (Examples: fish, horses, thimble, knitting needles, etc.) Present each hat to the group and ask the group to guess who it belongs to. Each person models his/her hat for the group.

TARGET ACTIVITY 12
Blessing Feathers

Goals

1. Encourage group participation.

2. Provide an opportunity to make a choice about what activity will be done.

3. Provide an opportunity for leadership (if appropriate).

Materials Needed

1. Drawing of turkey without tail feathers

2. Activity feathers — construction paper feathers with an activity written on them

3. Feathers with no writing on them

4. Easel to mount the picture of the turkey

5. Masking tape

6. Basket or box to put feathers in

7. Markers

Activity

1. Begin focusing group by singing traditional Thanksgiving songs: "Over the River and Through the Woods," "Now Thank We All Our God," and "We Gather Together." (Lyrics are on pages 41 and 42.)

2. Draw attention to the turkey: *This is supposed to be a picture of a turkey, but something is missing. Does anyone have any idea what it might be?* Encourage clients to respond.

3. Introduce the game "Blessing Feathers":

   a. Ask each client to share something he/she is thankful for or a blessing. Write this on a blank feather and encourage him/her to mount the feather on the turkey. Encourage all the clients to participate.

   b. After all the blessing feathers have been mounted, choose a client to pick an activity feather from a basket and read what it says to do, if appropriate; otherwise, the therapist will read it.

   c. Everyone does the activity and, if appropriate, the client who chose the feather will lead as much of the activity as possible.

   d. Encourage all the clients to choose an activity feather and participate in the activity. Suggested activities:

      1. Sing "Home, Sweet Home."

      2. Group dancing to "Turkey in the Straw."

      3. Parachute activity to a recording of "Sweet Georgia Brown."

      4. Wave small American flag to "My Country 'Tis of Thee."

      5. Play lummi sticks to a recording of "Shine On, Harvest Moon."

      6. Sing "America, the Beautiful."

4. Make a bulletin board from the finished "turkey" and display it in a location that the clients will be able to see. This activity also works well with an intergenerational group.

TARGET ACTIVITY 13
It's Raining...Again!

Goals

1. Encourage participation through discussion and song.

2. Promote weather awareness.

Materials Needed

1. "Rainy Day," *The Second Book of Children's Playsongs*, by Nordoff and Robbins (p. 9) or "Oh! What a Rainy Morning" sung to the tune of "Oh! What a Beautiful Morning." Chorus:

> Oh! What a rainy morning
> Oh! What a rainy day!
> There are so many things I'd
> Rather be doing today.

2. An umbrella

3. Four-leaf clover (see page 17)

4. Paper raindrops large enough to write on; two-dimensional paper umbrella

5. Easel and paper for mounting umbrella

6. Markers

7. Tape

Activity

1. Begin focusing the group by singing some "rainy day" songs. Examples: "Singing in the Rain," "It's Raining, It's Pouring," and "Rain, Rain, Go Away."

2. Display the umbrella. Keep it closed. (Clients usually become very agitated if an umbrella is opened inside: it represents bad luck.) Ask clients what this is used for.

3. Begin singing "Rainy Day" or "Oh, What a Rainy Morning." After singing the chorus, ask each client what he or she likes to do on a rainy day. Sing each response in the song using the music from the verse. Example:

> Ann would like to read a good book
> Howard would rather stay in bed
> Rosie and Bertha would have a cup of tea
> While Helen would bake a loaf of bread.

As each client tells what he or she likes to do on a rainy day, have a staff member write it on a "raindrop." Ask the client to put it on the paper umbrella. Or, mount the paper umbrella on a poster board and bring the umbrella to each person.

4. Weave in other songs or activities that are suitable for a rainy day. Examples:

   a. "I'm Looking over a Four-Leaf Clover" (See page 17.)

   b. "Side by Side" - Hold hands while you sing.

   c. Parachute activity - Use a balloon in the middle of the parachute. Encourage clients to make it "dance" by lifting and lowering the parachute.

   d. "Rain, Rain, Go Away"

   e. "April Showers"

   f. "Let a Smile be Your Umbrella"

5. End session by singing "Wait 'Til the Sun Shines, Nellie." (Lyrics are on page 61.)

Wait Till the Sun Shines, Nellie

Wait till the sun shines, Nellie,
And the clouds go drifting by,
We will be happy, Nellie,
Don't you cry.
Down lovers' lane we'll wander,
Sweethearts, you and I,
Wait till the sun shines, Nellie,
By and by.

Wait till the sun shines, Nellie,
And the grey skies turn to blue
You know I love you, Nellie,
'Deed I do.
We'll face the years together
Sweethearts, you and I
Wait till the sun shines, Nellie,
By and by.

TARGET ACTIVITY 14
Flag Day

Goals

1. Encourage participation through discussion and music.

2. Stimulate memories of the United States and the flag.

Materials Needed

1. Four sheets of paper with one letter of the word F-L-A-G written on each of them

2. Markers

3. Easel or board to mount papers on

4. Small American flags (enough for each client and staff participating in the session)

5. Patriotic music recordings

6. Strips of red and white paper with patriotic songs or activities written on them in blue marker

7. White stars with patriotic activities written in blue marker

Activity

1. Pick a client to hold a U.S. flag and ask everyone to stand (if possible) and say the "Pledge of Allegiance."

2. Lead the group in singing "My Country 'Tis of Thee."

3. Begin a discussion about the flag and what it stands for in our country. Ask questions like these:

   a. *What are some of the nicknames for the U.S. flag?* (Old Glory, Stars and Stripes)

   b. *What do the stars stand for?* (The 50 states of the U.S.A.)

c. *What do the red and white stripes stand for?* (The 13 original colonies)

d. *Who was supposed to have made the first flag for George Washington?* (Betsy Ross)

4. Direct the group to the word F-L-A-G. Look at one letter at a time. Ask the clients to give words beginning with that letter and that describe a symbol of or a feeling for the flag. Examples:

F	L	A	G
Friendship	Love	America	God
Fathers	Loyalty	All who fought	Generosity
Future	Light	for it	Grand
Freedom	Leader		
Fellowship			

5. Choose each client to pick one of the "stars" or "stripes" activities for the group to do. Encourage the client to be the leader of the activity (if appropriate). Activities could include:

   a. Sing "You're A Grand Old Flag" - Pass out a flag for everyone to wave as they sing the song.

   b. Sing "God Bless America."

   c. Sing "The Star Spangled Banner."

   d. Play a recording of Sousa's "Stars and Stripes Forever" — Hand out lummi or rhythm sticks and play together.

   e. Play a recording of "This Land is Your Land" — Have a balloon toss.

6. Close by singing "America the Beautiful."

Additional Activity

Make a bulletin board using the FLAG cards and the "stars" and "stripes" activities. Ask clients to choose pictures of scenic America to add for a collage.

AMERICA

My country 'tis of thee,
Sweet land of liberty, of thee I sing;
Land where my fathers died,
Land of the pilgrim's pride,
From every mountainside, let freedom ring.

My native country, thee,
Land of the noble free, thy name I love.
I love thy rocks and rills,
Thy woods and templed hills;
My heart with rapture thrills like that above.

Let music swell the breeze,
And ring from all the trees sweet freedom's song.
Let mortal tongues awake;
Let all that breathe partake;
Let rocks their silence break, the sound prolong.

Our fathers' God, to Thee,
Author of liberty, to Thee we sing.
Long may our land be bright
With freedom's holy light;
Protect us by Thy might, great God, our King!

Spin the Bottle

Goals

1. Encourage group participation.

2. Encourage leadership (if appropriate).

3. Give an opportunity to make a choice by selecting activity strips.

Materials Needed

1. Empty large, plastic soda pop bottle (preferably clear)

2. Colored vinyl tape

3. Activity strips—strips of paper with an activity written on each strip

4. Scissors

5. Markers

Activity

Prior to Activity

1. Clean out the bottle and secure cap.

2. Cut a door in the middle of the bottle large enough to reach a hand inside the bottle, with one side still attached.

3. Cover the cut edges of the door and bottle with the vinyl tape (to keep clients from being cut).

4. Move the door in and out of the bottle to make it more flexible.

5. Put activity strips inside the bottle.

Target Activity

1. Begin focusing clients by asking if they ever played "Spin the Bottle."

2. Place the bottle in the middle of the circle of clients. Spin the bottle. Ask how to play "Spin the Bottle."

3. When the bottle stops, take it to the person it is pointing to and ask him/her to pick an activity strip out of the bottle's door.

4. Ask the client to read what is on the strip (if appropriate). Do that activity and encourage the client to be the leader, or to sit with you as you lead everyone.

5. Continue spinning the bottle, allowing each client a turn. (If necessary, stop the bottle in front of those clients who have not had turns.)

Activity Ideas

1. Patriotic theme

   "God Bless America" - sing-along

   Pledge of Allegiance/"My Country 'Tis of Thee" - Ask all the clients to stand (if possible). The client who chose the activity holds a small American flag and leads everyone in the Pledge of Allegiance (if appropriate). At its conclusion, the therapist leads the group in singing "My Country 'Tis of Thee." (I usually do this a cappella.)

   "This Land is Your Land" - Begin singing the song and encourage everyone to stand and join hands. Encourage everyone to dance and sing together.

2. Potpourri of Fun

   "Hokey Pokey" - group dance

   "Moonlight Bay" - use giant stretchband for group movement

   "Let Me Call You Sweetheart" - group sing-along

   "I'm Forever Blowing Bubbles" - balloon toss

Variations

Decorate the bottle to represent a particular holiday or theme:

   a. Patriotic: red, white, and blue ribbons; flag stickers; stars

   b. Christmas: red and green ribbons or tape; Christmas tree stickers; stars

   c. Spring: pastel ribbons; flower and baby animal stickers

   d. St. Patrick's Day: green soda bottle; shamrock stickers

TARGET ACTIVITY 16
The Luck of the Irish

Goals

1. Encourage participation.

2. Give opportunity to make choices.

3. Encourage gross motor movement.

Materials Needed

Session I - Shamrock prints

1. Green nontoxic paint

2. Potato stamps - cut potatoes in half and carve four-leaf clovers in them or use shamrock-shaped sponges

3. Tapes and records of Irish music

4. Mural paper covering activity table

Session II

1. Shamrock prints mounted on green poster board

2. Big box to mount poster board on

3. Tapes and records of Irish music

4. Four-leaf clover picture puzzle (see page 17)

5. Activity strips

6. Beanbag

Activity

Session I: Making Shamrock Prints

You will need extra hands for this session.

1. Begin the session in the music circle. Sing a few Irish songs, ending with "McNamara's Band." Ask the clients to stand up and dance or march over to the activity table (if appropriate).

2. Sit clients at a comfortable distance from each other.

3. Hand out a potato stamp to each client. Take a stamp and dip it into the paint. Demonstrate how to press it onto the paper to make a shamrock. Go to each client and admire his/her handiwork. Play Irish music in the background and ask if anyone has ever found a four-leaf clover. Write each client's name by his/her shamrock.

4. Close by singing "My Wild Irish Rose."

Between Sessions I and II: Construct Shamrock Prints

1. Cut out a big shamrock shape for each client from his/her potato prints. Include as many of their stamped shamrocks as you can. (Make sure the client's name is on his/her own shamrock.)

2. Make activity strips. Glue one strip on each shamrock. Some could include the following:
    a. "That's an Irish Lullaby" - balloon toss
    b. "Danny Boy" - group sing-along
    c. "When Irish Eyes are Smiling" - group or partner dancing
    d. "McNamara's Band - guided instrumental activity
    e. "My Wild Irish Rose" - sing-along
    f. "Irish Washer Woman" - lummi stick activity
    g. "I'll Take You Home Again, Kathleen" - dance

3. Tape the shamrocks on a piece of green poster board.

4. Mount poster board on the side or top of a box.

Session II

1. Focus clients with singing "I'm Looking Over a Four-Leaf Clover." Use the picture puzzle (page 17). Do the activity once.

2. Bring the shamrock prints out to the middle of the circle. Carry it around and sing "I'm Looking Over a Four-Leaf Clover" again, substituting the clients' names for the leaves. As you sing the client's name, point to his/her shamrock. Example:

I'm looking over a four-leaf clover
That I overlooked before!
This one is Joe's, the second is Pam's,
The next ones are Mildred's, Henry's, and Ann's,
No need explaining the ones remaining
Are Harvey's, Jim's and Sam's.
I'm looking over a four-leaf clover
That I overlooked before!

3. Place the box on a chair. Read the songs on the shamrocks.

4. Demonstrate to the clients how to choose the activity they want by tossing the beanbag onto the shamrock with their choice written on it.

5. After each person has taken a turn, remove the chosen shamrock from the poster board so it won't be picked again.

6. Make a mural or bulletin board with the shamrock prints.

Music Toss

Goals

1. Encourage gross motor movement.

2. Give opportunity for decision making.

3. Encourage group participation.

Materials Needed

1. Ring Toss game - a wooden frame with 5 upright pegs. Each peg has a point value - 5, 10, 15, 20, and 25 (center peg).

2. Three rings (plastic or rubber)

3. Music Toss Card - a poster board divided into five categories that correspond to the point value of the pegs in the Ring Toss. Each point value category also represents a music category, with several selections listed in each category. (See page 71 for sample Music Toss Card.)

4. Easel or board for mounting the Music Toss Card.

Activity

1. Begin focusing the group by placing the Ring Toss in the middle of the circle.

2. Demonstrate to the clients how to toss the rings onto the pegs.

3. Next, point to the Music Toss Card. Match the music categories to the pegs that you "ringed" on your demonstration. For instance, peg 5 - dance; peg 10 - religious; peg 25 - sing-along. If a ring is placed on several pegs, choose a favorite category from the ones represented on the Music Toss Card. Then, choose one activity from the music category. Example: Peg 5 is ringed - Dance is the category. Activity chosen - "Chicken Dance."

   Everyone does the activity with you and then you choose a client to take the next turn. (Allow the client to lead the activity, if appropriate.)

Options

1. Laminate the Music Toss Card with only the point values marked on the poster board. Then write the categories and activities on the laminated surface with a marker or grease pencil. This way you can change the categories or activities without making up a new card.

2. Variation for lower functioning clients: Instead of writing the selections on the poster, mount a paper bag under each category by gluing a strip of velcro on the poster and the back of the bag. Write the selections on strips of paper and place them in the appropriate bag. When the client has tossed the rings, remove the bag that represents his/her choice. Let the client choose a slip of paper as his/her selected activity.

Music Toss Card

5 Dance	10 Religious	15 Patriotic	20 Instrument	25 Sing-along
"Chicken Dance"	"Old Time Religion"	"God Bless America"	Play to music	"Daisy, Daisy"
"Mexican Hat Dance"	"Amazing Grace"	"Star-Spangled Banner"	Lummi sticks	"She'll Be Comin' Round the Mountain"
Slow dance	"In the Garden"	"Yankee Doodle"	Play along with me	"I've Been Workin' on the Railroad"
Square dance	"Amen"	"America"	"The More We Get Together"	"Till We Meet Again"
"Alley Cat" dance	"Michael, Row the Boat"	"America the Beautiful"	"When the Saints"	"Moonlight Bay"
Conga dance	"Count Your Blessings"	"This Land is Your Land"	"Old MacDonald"	"Side by Side"

TARGET ACTIVITY 18
Going on a Picnic

Goals

1. Encourage group participation through music and discussion.

2. Encourage seasonal awareness.

Materials Needed

1. Several sheets of white paper

2. Markers

Activity

1. Begin focusing the group by singing two or three songs, such as these:

   a. "In the Good Old Summertime"

   b. "Yes, We Have No Bananas"

   c. "Meet Me in St. Louis"

2. If it's a sunny day, talk about things you can do on a hot, summer day. Encourage the clients to talk about things you can do with another person in the summer. If it's raining, talk about what you would like to do if it was a sunny day.

3. Sing the following lyrics using the tune "Did You Ever See a Lassie?"

   > Let's go on a picnic
   > A picnic, a picnic
   > Let's go on a picnic
   > Oh, what shall I bring?

Go around the circle and ask the clients what they each will bring to the picnic. Ask a program aide or another therapist to write down the responses on a piece of paper. Use one sheet of paper for each client. Hand each client his "picnic paper." After all the clients have responded, sing the song again and use their suggestions for the verses.

Example:

> Nancy will bring pickles
> And Tom will bring hot dogs
> George will bring tomatoes
> We're ready to go!

Feature each client when you sing his/her name and food. If possible, schedule this activity on a day when the clients will be having a picnic. They'll be ready to eat!

Option

Write each person's name and his/her food on a big piece of paper on an easel. Sing the song all at once, going all around the circle as each name is mentioned. Use these "verses" for the "this way and that way" part of the song.

Additional Activity

This can be a good intergenerational activity. Sit the children in a circle, face-to-face with the clients. As each one shares a food, it will provide opportunities for spontaneous interaction. Plan a picnic afterwards.

TARGET ACTIVITY 19
My Favorite Things

This activity works best with a small group, no larger than six clients.

Goals

1. Encourage group participation through music and discussion.

2. Stimulate long-term memory of past hobbies.

Materials Needed

1. Props that will stimulate past hobbies or experiences:

   a. rolling pin/cooking utensils
   b. aprons - cooking and carpenter
   c. tools
   d. musical instruments
   e. knitting needles/yarn
   f. pin cushion
   g. paint and brushes
   h. deck of cards
   i. bingo cards
   j. book
   k. travel brochures
   l. sports equipment
   m. toy boat
   n. bathing suit
   o. mounted stamps
   p. coins (in clear bag)
   q. shells

   Send a note to the families for suggestions or look at clients' charts for possible preferences.

2. Large basket(s) with handle or trays.

3. Easel with a large sheet of paper mounted on it.

4. Markers

5. Tape that has recordings of songs that pertain to the different props. Examples:

    a. "Take Me Out to the Ball Game" - ball

    b. "Moonlight Bay" - toy or model boat

    c. "In My Merry Oldsmobile" - toy or model car

    d. "I Could Have Danced All Night" - dancing shoes

    e. "Someone's in the Kitchen With Dinah" - train hat

    f. "Mairzy Doats" - stuffed or ceramic horse

    g. "Anchors Away" - sailor hat

    h. "How Much Is That Doggie in the Window?" - toy dog

    i. "I'm Lookin' Over a Four-Leaf Clover" - four-leaf clover or picture of one

6. Camera/film

Activity

Before the session, list the names of the clients down the left side of the mounted paper.

1. Sing "My Favorite Things" from "The Sound of Music." As you are singing the song, begin filling the basket with the props.

2. After the song is over, ask each client to pick something from the basket that he/she would need in order to do something that they would like to do. Play tape recorded music that reinforces hobby ideas and sing along softly (if appropriate). In addition, ask clients questions about what they have chosen, such as:

    a. *Do you like to use [prop]?*

    b. *When have you used it?*

    c. *Did you work by yourself or did someone work with you?*

    d. *Did you have a favorite place to do your hobby?*

While you are interacting with the clients, ask a program aide or another therapist to write down the comments on a piece of paper. If this is not possible, tape record the session.

3. After everyone has chosen something, direct their attention to the easel. Go down the list of clients' names and write their selection. Example: Bob likes sailboats, Jan likes reading, Alice likes music, etc.

When the list is complete, you will have a new verse for "My Favorite Things." Sing the new verse through for the clients, and add "these are a few of my favorite things" at the end of the list. Example:

Bob likes sailboats
Jan likes reading
Alice likes music
Jerry likes chocolate cake
John likes getting shaved by Hazel
These are a few of my favorite things.

Sing the song again, featuring the clients you are singing about. In addition, ask a program aide or another therapist to take a picture of each client holding his/her prop.

4. Close the session by singing some favorite songs of the clients.

Additional Activity

Make a scrapbook of your clients' "favorite things." Ask the clients' families to send in pictures that pertain to each person's hobbies (past or present, if applicable). Make captions from the comments that were recorded during the session and display each picture taken. After the scrapbook is completed, place it in a prominent spot within your facility for easy access to everyone.

TARGET ACTIVITY 20
Auld Lang Syne

Goals

1. Encourage seasonal awareness.

2. Encourage group participation through the music and discussion.

Materials Needed

1. Picture of New Year's baby and Father Time: mount on an easel by the calendars

2. Calendars: One of the year ending and one of the new year beginning

3. Seasonal music

4. Easel

Activity

1. Begin focusing clients by singing "Auld Lang Syne." Display calendar on easel. Identify that it is a calendar—a listing of all the days, weeks, and months that belong in this present year. Announce that this year is almost gone and a new year is about to begin. Point to the New Year's baby and Father Time pictures to reinforce the passing of another year.

Variation I: Higher-functioning Clients

Open the calendar and focus on each month from January to December, in sequential order. Highlight holidays that occur during each month and name factual tidbits from history that have also occurred. In addition, match appropriate songs and activities that also correspond with it. Pick one simple activity for each month (or season). Examples begin on page 78.

Variation II: Lower-functioning Clients

Develop a seasonal review in place of a monthly review.

a. Choose two or three musical activities for each season. Keep them simple.

b. Reinforce seasonal awareness by making a grab bag for each season. Choose items that stress weather changes and traditional holidays over historical dates, events, and people. Examples:

Winter - hat and mittens, long johns, winter boots, ice skates

Spring - silk flower bouquet, picture of birds or garden, garden trowel, packet of seeds, closed umbrella

Summer - sandals, men's bathing suit, small American flag, baseball glove, sea shells

Fall - ruler, toy school bus, silk autumn leaves, decorative harvest corn, small football

Additional Activity

Make a seasonal file box that is organized by the months of the year. Add activities and resources on file cards and categorize them under the appropriate month. Then when you want to promote seasonal awareness, you have all the information ready to use.

Events and Activities

EVENT/SEASON	HISTORICAL/SPECIAL	MUSICAL ACTIVITY
JANUARY		
• New Year's Day, 1/1 • Martin Luther King, Jr. born 1/15/29 • Winter, snow • Super Bowl • Mozart born 1/27/1756 • Elvis Presley born 1/8/35 • Jerome Kern born 1/27/1885	• Inauguration of president, 1/20 • Jan. 1, 1863, Lincoln gives Emancipation Proclamation • Hot Tea Month • Soup Month	• Lummi sticks to patriotic music • "We Shall Overcome" • "Let It Snow" • "Jingle Bells" • "Winter Wonderland" • "Love Me Tender"
FEBRUARY		
• President's Day, 3rd Monday • Groundhog Day, 2/2 • A. Lincoln born 2/12/1861 • G. Washington born 2/22/1732 • Valentine's Day, 2/14 • G. Rossini born 2/29/1792 • Ash Wednesday (sometimes in March)	• African American History Month • First adhesive mail stamp introduced, 2/15	• Patriotic music or activity (see Flag Day in June) • Love song/slow dances • Selections from Rossini's "The Barber of Seville"

EVENT/SEASON	HISTORICAL/SPECIAL	MUSICAL ACTIVITY
MARCH		
• Beginning of spring • St. Patrick's Day • Purim (sometimes in February) • Glenn Miller born 3/1/04	• 1876, Alexander Graham Bell sent a message to Mr. Watson on the telephone • Music In Our Schools Month	• Irish music • "When You Wore a Tulip" • "What Do You Do in the Infantry?" by Glenn Miller and the Army Air Force Band
APRIL		
• Easter (sometimes in March) • Passover (sometimes in March) • William Shakespeare born, 4/23/1564 • James Audubon born 4/26/1785 • Income Tax Day, 4/15	• National Garden Month • Secretaries Day, 3rd or 4th Wednesday • Earth Day, 4/22	• Sacred music - "Up From the Grave," "O Sacred Head, Now Wounded" • "Hava Nagila"
MAY		
• Mother's Day, 2nd Sunday • Memorial Day, 5/30 Celebrated 4th Monday • May Day, May 1st • Kentucky Derby	• Barbecue Month • Strawberry Month • Senior Citizens' Month • National Pet Week • Victory in Europe Day, 5/7/45 • Union Pacific & Central Pacific trains met in Utah, 5/10/1869	• "Home, Sweet Home" • "America the Beautiful" • "I've Been Workin' on the Railroad" • "M-O-T-H-E-R" • "Doggie in the Window" • May Pole dance • "My Old Kentucky Home"
JUNE		
• Father's Day • Flag Day, 6/14 • Summer begins, 6/21	• Dairy Month • Fresh Fruits and Vegetables Month • "Birthday" of Donald Duck, 6/9/34	• "Oh My Poppa" • "In the Good Old Summertime" • "You're a Grand Old Flag" • "Yes, We Have No Bananas"
JULY		
• Independence Day • Stephen Foster born, 7/4/1826	• July 4, 1776 - signing of the Declaration of Independence • First walk on the moon, 7/20/69 • First singing telegram, 7/28/33	• "Yankee Doodle" • "God Bless America" • "Take Me Out to the Ball Game" • Make up a singing telegram
AUGUST		
• Dog Days • Summer vacations	• Ice Cream Month • National Catfish Month	• "In the Good Old Summertime" • "Michael, Row the Boat Ashore"

EVENT/SEASON	HISTORICAL/SPECIAL	MUSICAL ACTIVITY
SEPTEMBER		
• Labor Day, 1st Monday • Rosh Hashanah • Yom Kippur (sometimes in October) • Back to school • Autumn begins • Grandparents Day, 2nd Sunday	• Piano Month • Chicken Month • Constitution signed, 9/5/1787	• "This Land Is Your Land" • Dance, the Hora • "Chicken Dance" • "School Days"
OCTOBER		
• Columbus Day, 10/12 • Halloween • Harvest	• Pasta Month • United Nations Day, 10/24 • Stock Market crashed, 10/29/29 • 1st demonstration of electric light bulb by Edison	• "Shine On, Harvest Moon" • Square dance to "Turkey in the Straw" • "It's a Small World"
NOVEMBER		
• Veterans Day, 11/11 • Thanksgiving • John Philip Sousa born 11/6/1854 • Scott Joplin born 11/24/1868	• American Music Week, 1st week • Aviation History Month • Armistice Day, 11/11/18 • Gettysburg Address delivered, 11/19/1863 • Assassination of John F. Kennedy, 11/22/63 • "Birthday" of Mickey Mouse, 11/18/28	• "We Gather Together" • "Over There" • "The Entertainer" • "Star and Stripes Forever" • Mickey Mouse Club theme song
DECEMBER		
• Hanukah begins (sometimes in November) • Winter begins • Christmas, 12/25 • Beethoven born 12/16/1770 • Mary Martin born 12/1/13	• Pearl Harbor Day, 12/7/41	• "My Dreydl" • "Skater's Waltz" • "It's Beginning to Look a Lot Like Christmas" • "Away in the Manger"

TARGET ACTIVITY 21
From Here to There

Goals

1. Motivate memories of previous traveling experiences.

2. Give opportunity to make choices.

3. Encourage group participation by going on an imaginary journey.

Materials Needed

1. Train and airline tickets; cardboard keys - enough for every client.

2. Large map of the United States, mounted on a wall or portable easel. If the map is laminated, mark the route with a bright whiteboard marker. If not, make a plastic overlay.

   a. Buy enough clear plastic to cover the U.S. map (try a fabric store).

   b. Lay it over the map and tape it to the top of the map.

   c. Mark the route with a bright whiteboard marker.

   d. Mount the map on the easel.

   e. Lift up the plastic and flip it over to the back of the map.

3. Slides of several famous landmarks and different states across the United States. Resources can include:

   a. Families of clients - Ask families to loan slides or negatives from previous travels of the clients.

   b. Libraries - Local schools and public libraries usually have slides of famous landmarks and national parks.

c. Smithsonian Institution (1000 Jefferson Dr., SW, Washington, D.C. 20004; 202-357-2700)

d. National Geographic Society has videos of the different regions and state and national parks across the United States. These may be available in your local school and public libraries. (See page 99 for address.)

e. Horizons Unlimited (See page 98 for address.)

4. Travel tape - a series of recordings that correspond with the visuals used in the journey. Pages 84 and 85 list a number of states and corresponding songs. If you use a video, it won't be necessary to make the travel tape unless it contains a narration soundtrack.

5. A recording of "Bon Voyage" from the musical "Around the World in Eighty Days"

6. Silk scarves

7. Several small snacks featuring regional cuisine (Refer to Step 9 in the Activity.)

8. Transportation props - toy train engine, airplane, and car (or photographs); train conductor's hat and airline flight attendant's hat

9. State or regional memorabilia - hats, pennants, paperweights, thimbles, silver charms, spoons, flags, postcards, mugs, T-shirts, dolls.

Activity

1. Begin focusing the group by singing "This Land is Your Land" and "America the Beautiful."

2. Invite the clients to join you in a journey across the United States. Look at the map of the United States. Ask questions like these:

    a. *What ocean borders the East Coast?* (Atlantic) *Have you ever been there?*

    b. *What ocean borders the West Coast?* (Pacific) *Have you ever been there? What is it like?*

    c. *What country borders the Northern United States?* (Canada) *Have you ever been there?*

    d. *What country borders the Southwestern United States?* (Mexico) *Have you ever been there?*

e. *How many states are in the United States?* (50)

3. Discuss different forms of transportation and decide which one will be used for the journey.

   a. As you name each category, hold up visual and physical props while singing a corresponding song.

      Example - "Would you like to go by..."

      ...train? Put on the conductor's cap. Call out "All Aboard!" Hold up a toy train engine (or a photo) and sing "I've Been Workin' on the Railroad."

      ...airplane? Put on a pilot's cap or a flight attendant's hat. Hold up a model airplane and sing "Come, Josephine, in My Flying Machine."

      ...car? Sit down in a chair and pantomime starting a car. Invite everyone to ride away with Lucile by singing "In My Merry Oldsmobile."

   b. Between each category, ask the clients if they had traveled that way (train, airplane, car) before. Also ask: *Did you enjoy it? Where did you go? Did you go by yourself? with family? friends? Was it a long trip?*

   c. Encourage clients to agree on one category. If the group is traveling by train or airplane, pass out tickets to each client. If everyone is traveling by car, pass out the cardboard keys.

4. To begin the journey, locate on the map the town or city where your facility is located. Mark it by pressing a large gold star (backed with silly putty) onto the map.

5. Suggest a travel route to the clients and ask for their opinions. Indicate on the map what states, historical landmarks, and national parks you will be traveling to on the "journey." Highlight the route with the plastic overlay.

6. Begin playing "Bon Voyage." Collect everyone's ticket or key and hand out the silk scarves to each client. Encourage them to wave good-bye as the journey begins.

7. Turn on the projector, dim the lights, and begin playing the travel tape. Be sure the slides and music are coordinated to feature the same state or landmark. Be a tour guide by supplying area history and folklore.

8. Ask the clients if they have ever visited these states or landmarks before. If someone begins sharing one of his/her experiences, pause the recording and encourage the reminiscing. Ask questions about the feelings he/she had during this experience.

9. Periodically stop and take a rest for a stretch and snack. Choose a snack that is specific to the region you are resting in. Examples:

   a. Midwest - sliced Wisconsin cheese or wheat crackers

b. Southeast - fruit cup (peaches, apples, and citrus fruits)

c. Southwest - nacho cheese dip with tortilla chips

d. Mid-Atlantic - seafood salad (or tuna fish) on toast triangles

10. If appropriate, examine souvenirs and memorabilia from the region where you have "stopped." Ask if anyone has collected pennants, matchbook covers, thimbles, or silver charms from a trip. Ask, *Did you have a favorite? What state or country was it from?*

11. As you reach the end of your journey, sing "Side by Side." Discuss coming home. Ask, *Were you sorry to see a trip end? Was it good to be home? Did anyone ever have a homecoming party for you?*

12. To close the session, say something like this: *It's exciting to go to new places and see different things, but just like Dorothy said to Toto in "The Wizard of Oz," "There's no place like home." Let's end our journey today by singing "Home, Sweet Home."*

Additional Activity for Higher-functioning Clients

Match the capitol to the states.

a. Cut out 1" x 8½" strips of paper. Write a capitol or state on each strip.

b. Seat clients at a round table.

c. Place ten capitols and their corresponding states on the table.

d. Match each capitol and state.

e. Repeat steps d and e until all fifty states are matched.

States and Corresponding Songs

New York - "New York, New York"; "Give My Regards to Broadway"; "East Side, West Side"

Pennsylvania - "Pittsburgh, Pennsylvania"; "Fight on State"

Delaware - "Oh, Our Delaware"

Georgia - "At a Georgia Camp Meeting"; "Ramblin' Wreck from Georgia Tech"

West Virginia - "Hail, West Virginia"; "Country Roads"

Virginia - "Carry Me Back to Old Virginny"

Kentucky - "My Old Kentucky Home"

North Carolina - "Carolina Moon"; "Carolina in the Morning"

South Carolina - "Step to the Rear"

Tennessee - "Tennessee Waltz"; "The Ballad of Davy Crockett"; "Chattanooga Choo Choo"

Louisiana - "Battle of New Orleans"; "Fight for L.S.U."

Mississippi - "Ol' Man River"; "Forward Rebels"

Ohio - "Beautiful Ohio"; "Across the Field"

Illinois - "Chicago"; "We're Loyal to You, Illinois"

Texas - "The Yellow Rose of Texas"; "The Eyes of Texas"; "Ol' Texas"

Alabama - "Oh! Susanna"; "Yea, Alabama"

Missouri - "St. Louis Blues"; "Meet Me in St. Louis"

Oklahoma - "Oklahoma" from the musical "Oklahoma"; "Boomer Sooner"

Hawaii - "Blue Hawaii"; "Hawaiian Wedding Song"

California - "California, Here I Come"; "Sons of Westwood"

Indiana - "Back Home Again in Indiana"

You can also use pioneer and Broadway tunes to fill in the gaps. Examples include:

"Sweet Betsy from Pike"

"Red River Valley"

"On Top of Old Smokey"

"God Bless America"

"My Country 'Tis of Thee"

"The Old Chisholm Trail"

"Pick a Bale of Cotton"

"Little Brown Jug"

"The Little Brown Church in the Vale"

TARGET ACTIVITY 22
A Beauty Pageant

Goals

1. Encourage group participation through discussion and song.

2. Give opportunity to make choices.

3. Motivate memories of previous experiences.

Materials Needed

1. Birthday crown - try to get an inexpensive one with artificial gems. You can usually find one at a party supply store.

2. Three grab bags - You can use a pillowcase or sack with a drawstring.

3. Items associated with beauty. Suggestions:

People

a. baby pictures of clients and staff - enlist the help of the clients' families and staff to provide a photo (if available)

b. hairstyles from the 1940s to the present

Places

a. postcards that have replicas of famous works of art or of seasonal scenery

b. large pictures of different houses (check real estate agencies)

c. large pictures of flowers and gardens

Things

a. original recordings of famous vocal artists (if possible, include artists from different musical styles for comparison and client preference)

b. fashion magazines from the 1940s to the present

    c. several pieces of jewelry, different models of toy cars and trucks

  4. Small display table positioned in front of the circle

  5. Recordings and props needed for corresponding activities

  6. Camera and film

Activity

1. Hold the birthday crown (serving as a tiara) and begin singing, "Here She is, Miss America" (or Mr. America).

2. Begin a discussion about defining beauty. Ask questions like these:

   a. *Some people say that beauty is only skin deep. Do you agree?*

   b. *Other people say that beauty is in the eyes of the beholder. Do you agree?*

   c. *Still other people say that handsome is as handsome does. Do you agree?*

3. Ask, *Is everything beautiful?* Begin singing "Everything Is Beautiful." Encourage the clients to join in.

4. Invite the client to a "beauty contest." Say something like, *Today we're going to have a beauty contest. Instead of judging beautiful women, we're going to judge what we like about people, places, and things.*

5. Introduce one of the grab bags.

   a. Tell the clients what category the items represent.

   b. Demonstrate how to choose an item and discuss likes and dislikes.

   c. Give everyone an opportunity to choose an item from the bag and comment on it.

   d. Lead the group in a corresponding activity. (See suggestions on page 88.)

   e. Display each item on a table in the front of the group. At the end of a category, have the clients vote on the item that they prefer the most. Put the other items back in the grab bag.

   f. After judging the three categories, move the table towards the group and display the winners. Take a picture of the winners and the judges.

   g. Close the session by singing "Beautiful Dreamer." (Lyrics are on page 89.)

Suggested activities to correspond with the beauty items:

People

1. Baby Pictures

   a. Sing "You Must Have Been a Beautiful Baby." Go around the group and frame everyone's face with a headless tambourine or an empty picture frame.

   b. Try matching baby pictures to the correct client or staff person.

2. Hairstyles - After comparing hairdos, pass out silk scarves and play a recording of "I'm Gonna Wash That Man Right Out of My Hair." Encourage everyone to "wash" (shaking motion) with silk scarves.

Places

1. Scenic postcards - Sing "Let It Snow" for a winter scene; "Autumn Leaves" for a fall scene; "By the Beautiful Sea" for a beach scene; "I'll Be With You in Apple Blossom Time" for a spring scene.

2. Gardens - Sing "Garden Party," "In the Garden," or "Tiptoe Through the Tulips."

Things

1. Fashions - Toss a balloon to a recording of "Button and Bows" or "Five Foot Two, Eyes of Blue."

2. Music styles - Listen to original recordings of several artists. Encourage the clients to voice their preferences.

Additional Activities

1. Ask a beauty consultant to come in and "make over" willing clients with makeup and a new hairdo.

2. Ask a barber to come in and shave willing clients with an electric razor. Some men might like a haircut or trim.

Beautiful Dreamer

Beautiful dreamer, wake unto me,
Starlight and dewdrops are waiting for thee;
Sounds of the rude world heard in the day,
Lull'd by the moonlight have all pass'd away!
Beautiful dreamer, queen of my song,
List while I woo thee with soft melody;
Gone are the cares of life's busy throng
Beautiful dreamer, awake unto me!
Beautiful dreamer, awake unto me!

Beautiful dreamer, out on the sea
Mermaids are chanting the wild lorelie;
Over the streamlet vapors are borne,
Waiting to fade at the bright coming morn.
Beautiful dreamer, beam on my heart,
E'en as the morn on the streamlet and sea;
Then will all clouds of sorrow depart,
Beautiful dreamer, awake unto me!
Beautiful dreamer, awake unto me!

TARGET ACTIVITY 23
Sound Poetry

Goals

1. Encourage group participation in making a background tape for a poem.

2. Motivate memories of past summers.

Materials Needed

1. Tape recorder, blank tape

2. Poem on the chosen topic

3. Illustrations or tracings of characters in the selected poem. Make several double-sided copies of each illustration.

    a. Sample poem: "It's Summertime" - by Cindy Cordrey

       It's summertime
       Take time to hear
       The wonders all around
       In the sky and on the ground
       Thunder rumbling in a storm
       Children waking in the morn
       The croaking of a frog
       The barking of a dog
       The chirping of a bird
       Cows mooing in a herd
       The bleating of a lamb
       Waves crashing in the sand
       It's summertime
       Time to slow down
       To capture all around
       The wonders in the sky and on the ground.

    b. Characters to illustrate: children yawning, frog, dog, bird, cow, lamb

4. Instruments needed to enhance the backgound tape. Examples:

    a. gong (thunder)

    b. suspended cymbal (crashing waves)

5. Easel plus a piece of blank poster board

Activity

1. Read the poem to the clients. Focus their attention on the characters by displaying the characters' pictures as they appear in the poem "It's Summertime."

2. Ask, *What sounds do you like to hear in the summertime? Is there one sound that you look forward to hearing every summer? What is it?* Encourage responses.

3. Say, *Let's put some sounds to the picture to make this poem sound like summertime.*

    a. Assign each client a sound that represents a character. Hand him/her a character picture as a visual prop. Try to put all the bird chirpers together, barking dogs together, etc.

    b. Lower-functioning clients might find more success in using the gong or substituting a wind chime for chirping birds.

    c. Rehearse each group in the order that the characters appear.

4. Choose a higher functioning client to read the poem. Assign a staff member to him/her to provide assistance, if necessary.

5. Turn on the tape recorder. Rehearse each group doing its part of the poem, with the therapist giving verbal and physical prompts as needed. Keep recorder running.

6. Do one more complete reading and performance. Stop the tape recorder.

7. Rewind the tape. While waiting for the tape, thank everyone for making the tape. Talk about who might like to hear it.

8. Listen to the final performance and enjoy it together.

Additional Activity

This works well as an intergenerational activity. Seat the children in front of the clients, assigning them to character groups as well. This activity also can be done with poems on other themes.

TARGET ACTIVITY 24
Grubbing Around

Goals

1. Motivate memories of gardening.

2. Motivate memories of occasions when the clients have received flowers.

3. Give opportunity to make choices.

4. Give opportunity to express preferred foods and herbs.

Materials Needed

1. Fresh bouquet of various aromatic flowers or a planter of forced bulb flowers (e.g., tulips, daffodils, hyacinths)

2. Gardening tools (e.g., hand cultivator, hand trowel, pruning shears)

3. Bite-sized pieces of fresh vegetables and fruits (Note: Check with dietary staff for appropriate selection.)

4. Veggie and fruit trivia questions (See Step 4 on page 93.)

5. Herb bags

   a. Place a small amount of a dried and crushed aromatic herb in a five-inch square of cheesecloth (e.g., garlic, chives, sweet basil, lavender, oregano, mint, sage, dill, rosemary, or thyme.)

   b. Lift the corners toward the center to create a small pouch.

   c. Tie a bright ribbon around the opening to seal the herb.

   d. Put a tag on each bag: side one - name of the herb; side two - a picture of the herb plant (obtain from seed catalog).

   e. Place the bags in a lightweight clay pot.

6. Taped recordings of "Yes! We Have No Bananas," "Scarborough Fair," and "Heather on the Hill"

7. Tape recorder

Activity

1. Begin focusing the clients by encouraging them to smell and touch a fresh bouquet of fragrant flowers. Blooming bulbs like tulips or hyacinths work well also.

    a. Discuss the different colors and textures of the flowers.

    b. Ask the clients questions like these: *What is your favorite flower? Which flowers do you like to smell? Did you ever have a flower garden?* Use garden tools as visual props.

2. Ask these two questions: *On what occasions have you given flowers? Been given flowers?* Use musical prompts, by singing songs related to special occasions, to encourage discussion and reminiscing. Examples include:

    a. birthday - "You Must Have Been A Beautiful Baby," "Happy Birthday to You"

    b. wedding anniversary - "Anniversary Song," "Put On Your Old Grey Bonnet"

    c. thank you - "Thanks for the Memories," "Count Your Blessings Instead of Sheep"

    d. funeral - "In the Garden," "Amazing Grace"

    e. fancy dances - "I Could Have Danced All Night," "After the Ball Is Over"

    f. a job well done - "For He's a Jolly Good Fellow"

    g. get well - "My Favorite Things"

3. Examine various fruits and vegetables.

    a. Offer cut-up vegetables and fruits to the clients. (Be aware of clients who might choke on hard vegetables or fruit.) While passing a tray around the group, softly play a recording of "Yes! We Have No Bananas."

    b. Discuss preferences of fruits and vegetables. Ask questions like these: *What is your favorite fruit? vegetable? Have you ever grown fruit trees or had a vegetable garden? Did you enjoy it? Was it a necessity?*

4. Play a brief veggie and fruit trivia game. Introduce it by saying something like this: *Let's see how good we are at identifying vegetables and fruits.* Trivia questions may include:

    Higher-functioning Clients

    a. *What fruit is a twosome?* pear

    b. *What fruit keeps the doctor away?* apple

    c. *What is the opposite of a "girl" berry?* boysenberry

d. *What is the opposite of a white berry?*   blackberry

e. *What berry rhymes with buckleberry?*   huckleberry

f. *What vegetable grows ears?*   corn

g. *What vegetable has eyes?*   potato

h. *What vegetable will never get lost because it always "shows up"?*   turnip

i. *What vegetable can be crowded and crushed?*   squash

Lower-functioning Clients - complete the phrase

a. green...beans

b. lima...beans

c. navy...beans

d. green bell...peppers

e. bibb...lettuce

f. Bing...cherries

g. navel...oranges

h. Red Delicious...apples

i. Bartlett...pears

j. Harvard...beets

k. Concord...grapes

l. hazel...nuts

m. black...walnuts

n. wax...beans

o. new...potatoes

5. Discuss and identify various common herbs.

   a. Begin by asking clients, *Did you grow herbs in your flower or vegetable garden? Why?* Some answers might include: beautiful plants, repel unwanted insects, entice helpful insects.

   b. Pass around the clay flower pot holding the herb bags. Begin recording of "Scarborough Fair" and "Heather on the Hill."

   c. Encourage the clients to choose a bag and smell it.

   d. Ask the clients for ways the different herbs can be used (e.g., cooking, sachets for pleasant-smelling linens, old-time remedies).

6. Close the session by singing "All Things Bright and Beautiful." (Lyrics are on page 96.)

Additional Activities

1. Ask the activities department to coordinate these activities:

   a. Start seeds for spring planting.

   b. Make vegetable soup.

   c. Paint and stencil clay pots.

2. Hold a "Flower Pot Sing-along":

   a. Write the titles of favorite sing-along songs on slips of pastel paper.

   b. Pass the pot around the music circle.

   c. Let each client choose a song for the group to sing.

All Things Bright and Beautiful

All things bright and beautiful,
All creatures great and small,
All things wise and wonderful,
The Lord God made them all.

Each little flower that opens,
Each little bird that sings,
He made its glowing colors,
He made its tiny wings.

The tall trees in the green wood,
The pleasant summer sun,
The ripe fruits in the garden,
He made them, every one.

He gives us eyes to see them,
And lips that we may tell
How great is God Almighty,
Who has made all things well.

Resources for Developing Target Activities

Therapeutic Resources

Activities and Approaches for Alzheimer's, by Sally Freeman, 134 Greenwood Ave., Decatur, GA 30030.

Down Memory Lane, by Beckie Karras, ElderSong Publications, P.O. Box 74, Mt. Airy, MD 21771; 800-397-0533.

The Lost Chord, by Melanie Chavin, ElderSong Publications, P.O. Box 74, Mt. Airy, MD 21771; 800-397-0533.

Harvest of Holidays, Collier's Junior Classics Series, Crowell-Collier Publishing Co., 866 Third Ave., New York, NY 10022.

Sense Up, by Zoe Ann Dearing and Maria Ciolfi, Therapeutic Services Dept., Jewish Center for the Aged, Chesterfield, MO 63017.

Periodicals

"Creative Forecasting," 2607 Farragut Circle, Colorado Springs, CO 80907; 719-633-3174. A monthly publication for activity professionals.

"ElderSong - The Music and Gerontology Newsletter," Beckie Karras, Editor, ElderSong Publications, P.O. Box 74, Mt. Airy, MD 21771; 800-397-0533.

"Reminisce," 5927 Memory Lane, P.O. Box 998, Greendale, WI 53129-9915. Bimonthly publication focusing on the "good old days."

Collections of Popular Music - Past and Present

Best Loved Songs of the American People, by Denes Agay, Doubleday and Company, 1540 Broadway, New York, NY, 10036. This collection of songs deals with America in colonial times, then progresses through American history to the 1970s. Includes notes on the songs with a brief summary about the composer and the song's time period.

The Fireside Book of Favorite American Songs, Simon and Schuster, Inc., Rockefeller Center, New York, NY 10020.

The Golden Book of Favorite Songs, Hall and McCreary Company, Chicago, IL.

Reader's Digest Songbooks, Reader's Digest Association, Inc., Pleasantville, NY 10570; 800-431-1246.

- Children's Songbook
- Country Western Songbook
- Family Songbook
- Family Songbook of Faith and Joy
- Festival of Popular Songs
- Unforgettable Musical Memories
- Merry Christmas Songbook
- Popular Songs That Will Live Forever
- Remembering Yesterday's Hits
- Treasury of Best Loved Songs

EQUIPMENT RESOURCES

Instrumental

Suzuki Musical Instrument Corporation, P.O. Box 261030, San Diego, CA 92126; 800-854-1594.

Richmond Music Center, Ltd., 243 Main Street, Staten Island, NY 10307; 718-967-4686.

Rhythm Band, Inc., P.O. Box 126, Fort Worth, TX 76101-0126; 800-424-4724.

The World of Peripole, Inc., P.O. Box 146, Brown Mills, NJ 08016; 800-443-3592.

Recordings, Tapes, Parachutes, Videos, Props

Hammatt Senior Products, P.O. Box 727, Mt. Vernon, WA 98273; 206-428-5850.

Kimbo Educational Resources, P.O. Box 477H, Long Branch, NJ 07740; 800-631-2187.

Horizons Unlimited, Geriatric Educational Corp., 27 East Front Street, Media, PA 19063; 215-566-6248. Provides members with kits containing props and memorabilia about a specific event or topic. Kits can be rented on a weekly or monthly basis. No training is necessary to obtain the kits, but training is available for a fee. Reservations for a specific kit need to be requested in advance to ensure availability.

National Geographic Society, 1145 17th Street, NW, Washington, DC 20036; 800-638-4077.

Oriental Trading Company, P.O. Box 3407, Omaha, NE 68103-0407; 800-228-2269. Catalog of inexpensive seasonal decorations and props.

GENERAL REFERENCE BOOKS

Austin, Barbara. 1988. *Alzheimer's Family Handbook.* Visiting Nurse Association of Metropolitan Atlanta, Inc.

Batcheller, John, and Monsour, Sally. 1972. *Music in Recreation and Leisure.* Dubuque, IA: Wm. C. Brown Company Publishers.

The History of Our United States. 1990. Pensacola, FL: A Beka Book Publishing.

Levin, Gail; Levin, Herbert D.; and Safer, Nancy D. 1975. *Learning Through Music.* Boston, MA: Teaching Resources Corporation.

Mace, Nancy, and Rabins, Peter V., M.D. 1981. *The 36-Hour Day: A Family Guide to Caring for Persons with Alzheimer's Disease, Related Dementing Illnesses and Memory Loss in Later Life.* Baltimore, MD: Johns Hopkins University Press.

Volicer, Ladslav; Fabizewski, Kathy; Rheaume, Yvette; and Lasch, Kathryn. 1988. *Clinical Management of Alzheimer's Disease.* Rockville, MD: Asen Publishers, Inc.

Williams, Janice L., and Downs, Janet. 1984. *Educational Activity Programs for Older Adults: A 12 Month Idea Guide for Adult Education Instructors and Activity Directors in Gerontology.* New York, NY: The Haworth Press, Inc.

ABOUT THE AUTHOR

Cindy Cordrey is a Certified Music Therapist-Board Certified who has worked with various special needs populations since 1982. In 1987, she became a music therapy consultant for an Alzheimer's adult day treatment facility in Wilmington, Delaware, where she currently is employed. Cindy also conducts workshops for local caregiver support groups.

Other Resources Published By ElderSong Publications

Down Memory Lane

With a Smile and a Song: Singing With Seniors

Moments To Remember

Mind Stretchers

Trivia Treasury: Trivia and Word Games for Older Adults

I Hear Memories!

Funny Bones Don't Get Arthritis: Humor for the Young at Heart

What Do You Know? Trivia Fun and Activities for Seniors

The Lost Chord: Reaching the Person with Dementia through the Power of Music

Barbers, Cars, and Cigars: Activity Programming for Older Men

Mind Joggers

Hooray For Hollywood: Trivia and Puzzles for those Today Who Remember Yesterday

Musings, Memories, and Make Believe

Puzzlers, Volumes 1 and 2

"Eldersong: The Music and Gerontology Newsletter"